Practical Guide to Geriatric Medication

SO-BIF-087

RC 953.7 .P72

Practical guide to geriatric medication

Practical Guide to Geriatric Medication

Medical Economics Company **MEBD** Book Division
Oradell, New Jersey 07649

RC
953.7
.P72

Library of Congress Cataloging in Publication Data

Main entry under title:

Practical guide to geriatric medication.

    1.   Geriatric pharmacology—Addresses, essays,
lectures. I. Burant, Ralph J. [DNLM: 1. Geriatrics.
WT100 P8955]
RC953.7.P72   615'.7   80-13682
ISBN 0-87489-205-8

Design by Susan Sonkin

ISBN 0-87489-205-8

Medical Economics Company
Oradell, New Jersey 07649

Printed in the United States of America

Copyright © 1980 by Litton Industries, Inc. Published by Medical Economics Company,
a Litton division, at Oradell, N.J. 07649. All rights reserved. None of the content of this
Litton publication may be reproduced, stored in a retrieval system, or transmitted in any form
or by any means (electronic, mechanical, photocopying, recording, or otherwise) without the
prior written permission of the publisher.

Contents

Contributors to This Book   vii

Foreword   ix

Acknowledgments   xxi

Chapter **1 Drug Therapy in the Elderly**   **1**
Morton Ward, M.D., and Morris Blatman, R.Ph.

The pluses and minuses of eight drug
administration routes   26

Chapter **2 How Aging Alters the Actions of Drugs**   **27**
Zachary I. Hanan, R.Ph., M.S.

Physiology of the elderly   30

How orally administered drugs
get into the bloodstream   34

Dehydration in elderly patients   36

Chapter **3 How Psychotropic Drugs Can Go Astray**   **43**
Marc Bachinsky, R.Ph., M.S.

Guide to adverse effects of psychotropic drugs
in the elderly   46

Problems of simple aging   54

Recognizing causes of aberrant behavior   56

Chapter **4 Tailoring Cardiovascular Therapy
to the Patient**   **59**
Fred S. Gordon, R.Ph., M.S.

Chapter **5 OTC Drugs and the Elderly**   **71**
Peter P. Lamy, Ph.D.

Major OTC/Rx drug interactions   74

Salicylate influence on some lab test values   80

Salicylate/Rx drug interactions   86

Chapter **6 Medication Mistakes and Noncompliance**   **93**

Foods that foil drugs   96

Crushing tablets, opening capsules:
When is it safe?   104

A prescriber's checklist   134

Chapter **7 Nutrition in the Elderly:
Practical Recommendations**   **139**
Myron Winick, M.D.

Partial list of common drugs affecting vitamin
levels in the elderly   149

Marc Bachinsky, R.Ph., M.S., is assistant director of pharmaceutical services for University Hospital, The State University of New York at Stonybrook.

Eleanor Bauwens, R.N., Ph.D., is associate professor and associate dean for the baccalaureate program in the College of Nursing at the University of Arizona, Tucson.

Morris Blatman, R.Ph., is on the pharmaceutical staff at the Philadelphia Geriatric Center.

Ann Boylan, R.N., M.A., is instructor of nursing, inservice education, at the Ruth Taylor Geriatric and Rehabilitation Institute, Hawthorne, N.Y.

Cindy Clemmons, R.N., B.S.N., is assistant director of inservice at Citizens Memorial Hospital, Victoria, Tex.

James C. Cope, M.D., who wrote the foreword, is retired from his practice in internal medicine, and lives in Rocheport, Mo.

Gilles L. Fraser, R.Ph., formerly pharmacist at the Central Maine Medical Center, Lewiston, is a D.Pharm. candidate in the School of Pharmacy at the University of Minnesota, Minneapolis.

Fred S. Gordon, R.Ph., M.S., is assistant director of pharmaceutical services at Mercy Hospital, Rockville Centre, N.Y.

Zachary I. Hanan, R.Ph., M.S., is director of pharmaceutical services at Mercy Hospital, Rockville Centre, N.Y.

Peter P. Lamy, Ph.D., is professor and director of institutional pharmacy programs and chairman of Pharmacy Practice and Administrative Science at the University of Maryland School of Pharmacy, Baltimore.

Keith Lerner, R.Ph., who was a student when he helped with the research for chapters 2, 3, and 4, is now a practicing pharmacist and is studying for his M.B.A. at the University of Syracuse.

Bernard Marbach, M.D., is medical director at the Ruth Taylor Geriatric and Rehabilitation Institute, Hawthorne, N.Y.

Henry A. Palmer, Ph.D., is assistant dean for clinical affairs in the School of Pharmacy at the University of Connecticut, Storrs.

Morton Ward, M.D., is medical director of the Philadelphia Geriatric Center.

Myron Winick, M.D., is director of the Institute of Human Nutrition at Columbia University's College of Physicians and Surgeons, New York, N.Y.

According to recent estimates, 80 per cent of people over 60 have a chronic disease, and of those, 35 per cent have three or more such conditions. The simultaneous treatment of multiple diseases provides fertile ground for drug incompatibilities and patient confusion over instructions for taking multiple medications. And when concurrent diseases are treated by different doctors, the possibility for excessive medication by drugs of similar actions increases as do the chances for incompatible combinations. Instructions from several doctors may also confuse patients.

Those are just a few of the complex problems that health-care professionals who work with elderly patients face. This book brings together discussions of a whole range of such problems and should prove helpful to all physicians, nurses, pharmacists, physician assistants, nurse practitioners, and staffs of health-care facilities that serve the elderly. But it should also prove helpful to noninstitutional physicians and other professionals. Because it was my own kind of work, I'd like to reflect on some of the more common problems that primary-care physicians in private practice see almost every day. Let's imagine what can happen to an older person during the course of treatment:

Mrs. Smith, 82, is sitting in front of the doctor listening to his pronouncement while he writes the inevitable prescription. "I don't find much wrong but a little high blood pressure. Take this medication and let me see you again in two weeks."

Mrs. Smith knew she had a little problem with high blood pressure; another doctor had told her that. She had come for a pain in the back, which she didn't get an opportunity to mention. Just as she was about to bring it up, the doctor had whisked out of the room and left her to his assistant.

Mrs. Smith also wanted to ask exactly how she was to take the medicine. She didn't get the chance. At the drugstore, she didn't talk at all to the pharmacist, as she had intended. A clerk took her prescription and in a while handed her back a bottle of unimpressive white pills with no distinguishing features. She asked about instructions and was told that they were written on the bottle.

At home she got out her magnifying glass and found that the curved surface of the bottle would allow only one letter of the label instructions at a time to come into focus. She finally puzzled out the words "one tablet four times a day." It didn't say before, after, or during meals or whether to get up in the middle of the night to take one. She decided to take them every six hours, at 6 A.M., noon, 6 P.M., and midnight.

Mrs. Smith took a pill with her dinner but missed the midnight dose because she forgot to set the clock. To make up for it, she took two the next morning. By the time she had taken another at noon and a third dose at 6 P.M., the bottle got so shuffled around in the medicine cabinet that she wasn't sure she was taking the correct medication. She was careful to take a white pill that looked the same, but she didn't want to go to the bother of using the magnifying glass to make sure. For months she had intended to clean out the medicine cabinet but hadn't gotten around to it; it held all the medicine bottles she had collected since she moved into her apartment three years ago.

In addition to her new medicine, Mrs. Smith was also taking three other medications from another doctor several times a day on a different schedule. She gave no thought to the possibility that there might be some difficulty taking all of those pills together. It was inconceivable to her that doctors would give her anything harmful.

On her next visit, Mrs. Smith was able to talk about her backache, which she still had. The doctor gave her another prescription. This time, just like the last, the assistant had her out in the hall before she was able to ask about it. She didn't go to the drugstore. She took the prescription home and put it in her desk. She was irked with the physician and refused to take the medicine.

Mrs. Smith's case makes it clear that knowing the pharmacology of a drug and how to write a prescription for it isn't all that's needed for the proper treatment of an older person.

The physician may think only of what the medicine will do for his patient's condition after it has been correctly taken and absorbed. To the patient, taking medication may be much more complex. It's a constant reminder that disease exists, that something is wrong. It can remind others that the patient is ill, perhaps dying, and needs more love and care.

Every physician has had the experience of finding that a patient of his now and then takes medication that was prescribed years ago by some physician for reasons that have long since been forgotten. The ritual of taking pills seems to have some significance on its own, aside from pharmacology. I've seen instances in my own practice in which I was sure that, for the patient, taking medicine was equivalent to taking the sacrament of Communion. For those reasons, it can sometimes be extremely difficult to take a person off a medication.

At my request, one of my patients once brought to the office all the medicines he was accustomed to taking, even if only now and then. They added up to 16 different drugs that he'd managed somehow to have refilled through the years. With further questioning, I found that he was also taking at least as many more nonprescription items that he didn't consider to be medicine, since he could buy them over the counter. It may be difficult to break such drug patterns. Many older persons may have developed dependencies on drugs and experience all kinds of symptoms, usually imaginary, when they are stopped.

At the other extreme, refusal to take medication is another problem that physicians may discover now and then. Some patients take pleasure in refusing to do anything their children or their caretakers want them to. Even if an attendant succeeds in putting a pill in the patient's mouth, it's not certain that it will get to the stomach or to the bloodstream.

While it's referred to only tangentially in this book, one of the most important decisions in patient care is whether to medicate at **xiii** all. The mere presence of a disease is not a reason for prescribing a drug. Its side effects may be worse than the disease.

A California study of drug therapy in skilled nursing facilities found that, too frequently, drugs were used to treat the adverse effects of other drugs and that, while drugs were frequently added to regimens, they were only rarely deleted.

A striking example of drug overload that the researchers of this study came upon was described in *Pharmacy Management*, March-April 1979:

"For example, one patient had an anti-inflammatory drug added to his daily regimen of sodium salicylate. This led to complaints of epigastric distress, for which he was administered Donnatal. The anti-inflammatory drug was also the probable cause of early morning frontal headaches and dizziness, for which he was given APC with codeine and Antivert, respectively. The codeine, of course, led to complaints of constipation, so a daily stool softener and a laxative were added to his drug intake. For good measure, he was given thrice-weekly shots of vitamin B_{12} and B-complex in each buttock. For each new complaint, the patient was given another drug, which in turn led to yet another new complaint.

"So, this 'chronic complainer,' whose only problem a short time ago had been early morning stiffness, now suffers from stomach discomfort, headaches, dizziness, diarrhea or constipation (depending on which drug was taken most recently), and local discomfort from 'all those shots.'"

Elderly patients look for freedom from symptoms, and not necessarily cure. A person older than 90, taking medication for arthritis and diverticulosis, is probably not made more comfortable by treatment for minimal hypertension, but may be made worse by some side effect. Unless cure is easily attained—unlikely with the degenerative diseases of old age—the aim of treatment should be comfort. This is as true of the potentially fatal diseases as it is of the less serious.

I've seen patients who were living comfortably with a slow-growing carcinoma made miserable by chemotherapy which was not intended to cure and did not palliate. I once treated an elderly physician and his wife, both of whom had cancer. His was colon cancer, while hers was a fibrous cancer of the breast. For some reason, both refused to countenance the fact that they had cancer and therefore refused treatment. Both lived happily and comfortably for several years only to die of something else. In retrospect, they were both wiser than I was. There was nothing we could have done to make either of them happier or more comfortable.

When a decision to treat has been reached, the first thing to determine is whether the patient can take the medication indicated. It's essential to ask about adverse reactions. Many patients have had bad experiences with one or more medications, which perhaps convinced them that they can't tolerate these drugs. Even if this sensitivity is wholly psychological in nature, it nonetheless is very real to the patient. When a patient says he can't take a medication, it shouldn't be prescribed.

Having determined that there will be no predeterminable adverse reactions, the next step is to find out what other drugs the patient is taking. This may mean that the patient has to make an additional trip to the office bringing all his medications, because the wise doctor wants to see for himself what drugs the patient is using. The number, variety, and age of some of these preparations can be amazing. At this point, it's good to cut down on the number of pills the patient is taking. Many complaints often disappear when the drug load is reduced.

Next, the patient is instructed how to take the medicine. Every four hours or three times a day is not definite. After or before meals, or during meals and at bedtime is a better way of making the instructions stick. Linking the time of medication to other routine activities will usually result in better-timed medication and a minimum of skipped doses. Chapter 6 of this book has many suggestions for assuring patient compliance.

It's a good idea to prescribe just enough medication to last until the next visit. If this is done and the patient is instructed to bring the bottle with him on the next visit, the physician can see whether the instructions have been followed. If the patient is given 30 pills and told to take one with meals and at bedtime, he should have two left when he visits the physician again in a week.

It's also important to tell the patient to take all of the medicine that's prescribed. Some patients stop medications when the symptoms subside. If this is not what the doctor wants, he should give firm instructions about taking all the medicine that is dispensed. Such a policy keeps bottles from accumulating in the medicine cabinet, which can foster self-medication with old drugs, at a time when they might be contraindicated.

Many older persons consider themselves authorities concerning their favorite remedies. Unless there's some reason for not doing so, it's just as well to let these patients carry on with them, so long as these preparations are innocuous. This leaves these patients with at least the feeling of control over their own bodies, a feeling that many older persons cherish. By allowing this latitude in things that aren't important, it may be much easier to get cooperation in the areas that matter more.

Those are just a few of the problems that the primary-care physician who treats geriatric patients should be aware of. The remainder of this book deals at length with particular problems of geriatric medication, offering insights, theory, and fact along with practical suggestions for the wide range of health-care professionals who deal with drugs for the elderly.

A final point: Some nursing homes have wisely instituted the practice of drug-free days for their residents. Patients in these facilities, as do most elderly patients, take many medications, and it takes these medications a long time to pass through their systems. The results of this drug holiday are no loss of therapeutic effect of medications, and a decreased incidence of adverse side effects.

If there were some way to monitor the compliance of elderly patients who are not in institutions so that they wouldn't get careless in their drug routines after having drug-free days, it would be good to try this idea with them, too.

James C. Cope, M.D.
Rocheport, Missouri

Acknowledgments

"Drug Therapy in the Elderly" originally appeared in the February 1979 issue of *American Family Physician* (copyright © 1979 by *American Family Physician*). The box that accompanies it appeared in the January 1978 *RN*.

"How Aging Alters the Actions of Drugs" was the first of a three-part series on geriatric medications in *RN* Magazine. This installment appeared in the January 1978 issue. One of the accompanying boxes appeared in the same issue with it. The other, "Physiology of the elderly," is from *Drug Topics*, July 1, 1974. The section on dehydration is an excerpt from the August 1979 issue of *RN*.

"How Psychotropic Drugs Can Go Astray," the second of the *RN* series, appeared in the February 1978 issue. The guide to adverse effects of these drugs was published with it. The other two boxes are from the June 1975 *Hospital Physician*.

"Tailoring Cardiovascular Therapy to the Patient," from the March 1978 *RN*, concluded that magazine's geriatric medications series.

"OTC Drugs and the Elderly" and the boxes that accompany it appeared in the November 1979 issue of *Current Prescribing*.

Much of the material in "Medication Mistakes and Noncompliance" comes from studies and brochures developed as parts of a Roche Laboratories program in medication education for elderly patients. Several of the memory aids suggested in that chapter come from "Teaching the Elderly to Avoid Accidental Drug Abuse," by Charlotte Isler, R.N., which appeared in the November 1977 *RN*. The accompanying "Foods that foil drugs," is from the September 1978 *RN*. The table on crushing tablets and opening capsules first appeared in the August 1978 *RN*. It was greatly expanded by the authors for inclusion in this volume.

"Nutrition in the Elderly" is from the September 1978 *Current Prescribing*. The accompanying box is from the September 15, 1978, *Drug Topics*.

The book was compiled and edited by Ralph J. Burant of the Medical Economics Company Book Division staff.

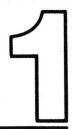

Drug Therapy in the Elderly

By Morton Ward, M.D., and Morris Blatman, R.Ph.

The elderly are the fastest growing segment of our population. The number of Americans over age 65 has been growing at a rate three times faster than that of the general population. In 1940, men and women age 65 and older represented less than 7 per cent of the total population; by 1970, that figure had risen to about 10 per cent, or more than 20 million. Between 1900 and 1960, the general population doubled but the number of persons over 65 quadrupled. Projections indicate that there will be 27.5 million people over age 65 by 1990.

Judge and Caird, in their book *Drug Treatment of the Elderly Patient*, state that 12 per cent of the British population is older than age 65 and accounts for 33 per cent of the expenditure of the National Health Service and an equivalent proportion of the drug bill. They

1

also state that approximately one-sixth of the older people take three or more drugs per day. There is evidence that the situation in the United States is similar to that in Great Britain. It's urgent, then, that physicians and other health-care personnel understand the effects of drug therapy in the elderly, because the potential for harm is greatest in older patients.

Concepts based on drug therapy of the mature adult are not applicable to the elderly. Drug dosage is usually reduced in older patients. With aging, the amount of fat relative to lean body mass increases. This fact and the relative intolerance of the elderly to drugs, though the exact mechanisms for these changes aren't clear, have been cited as reasons for drug dosage reduction.

Multiple concurrent disease processes are a constant invitation to use more and larger doses of drugs to control symptoms and manage the disturbed behavior that tends to accompany acute illness. The chance of a drug reaction or interaction rises dramatically with an increase in the number of drugs being taken.

At any one time, 40 to 55 per cent of the beds in acute-care hospitals are occupied by patients older than age 65. Studies on patient exposure to potentially noxious agents during a hospital stay have revealed an alarmingly high number of such drugs. The elderly have a reduced tolerance for such an onslaught; they're more at risk of overdosage and untoward effects than younger people.

DRUG-INDUCED CHANGES IN ABSORPTION

The ability to absorb substances in the upper gastrointestinal tract is unchanged in the elderly. However, absorption is affected by changes in transit time and the formation of insoluble complexes in the small intestine. Drugs that slow gastrointestinal motility increase the time available for absorption and therefore intensify the drug effect. Such drugs include anticholinergics, tricyclic antidepressants, phenothiazines, and antihistamines. Drugs that increase gastrointestinal motility or cause diarrhea decrease absorption and therefore reduce the drug effect; this is particularly true of preparations intended for prolonged or delayed release.

In the presence of calcium or iron salts, tetracycline forms insoluble metal complexes. The net effect is a significant decrease in the amount of tetracycline absorbed. Since anemia occurs in about 20 per cent of older patients, the use of iron in this group is probably considerable. Even when the iron is discontinued, there is quite a delay before the bowel is substantially clear of iron salts. Antacids containing calcium or aluminum should also be avoided during the administration of tetracycline.

DRUG
DISPLACEMENT

A significant mechanism of drug interaction is the displacement of one drug by another from protein-binding sites. Increased amounts of the displaced drug will then be present in the free state and will exert a marked and unexpected effect. Salicylates and phenylbutazone (Azolid, Butazolidin), for example, have been shown to displace tolbutamide and increase its hypoglycemic effect. Since the incidence of diabetes rises with age, the likelihood of such an occurrence is considerable.

Although anticoagulant therapy must always be approached carefully in the elderly, venous thrombosis, pulmonary embolism, and arterial embolism are definite indications for its use. A number of drugs, including phenylbutazone, clofibrate (Atromid-S), and chloral hydrate, may displace warfarin (Coumadin, Panwarfin) and result in an increased anticoagulant effect.

There's evidence that these types of displacement effects are more prevalent in the elderly and that their consequences may be more severe.

PATIENT-RELATED
PROBLEMS

Many problems with elderly patients stem from difficulties in communication. Vision and hearing are frequently impaired in older people. The physician must be sure that his message has not only reached the proper receptors but has traveled on, registered, and is fully understood. Attention span is limited, so the physician should avoid drawn-out, complicated instructions. The physician should, of course, give oral instructions on drug use, but these should be reinforced with written directions so that the patient or a member of the family can check the note, the patient's interpretation, and the label on the container.

A significant number of drug errors are made by skilled person- nel in institutions, so it's not difficult to imagine the possibilities for error when an older person with visual problems and impaired mem- ory tries to self-administer a drug regimen like the following: digoxin once daily; Lasix daily in the morning; a potassium supplement (to be dissolved in water) three times a day; Valium twice a day; iron three times a day, after meals; and chloral hydrate one-half hour before bedtime.

The fact that certain medications have been prescribed doesn't warrant the assumption that the patient is actually taking them. In our skilled nursing facility, where drugs are administered by a nurse whose instructions are to wait until the medication is in the patient's mouth, a female patient was found to have a collection of at least 250 pills and capsules of all sizes, colors, and shapes. All of them lacked the shiny manufacturers' finish as a result of a brief time in the patient's mouth.

In this instance, the woman was doing fine, so I suspect that her judgment with respect to the medication was probably better than her physician's. However, I also remember more serious situations when, as an intern, I rode an ambulance and picked up patients at their homes. Once, after moving the bed to transfer an elderly patient in pulmonary edema, I found a sizable collection of digitalis tablets where the bed had been.

CONSIDERATIONS IN
PRESCRIBING DRUGS

Medications that aren't clearly indicated should be avoided. There are many drugs whose efficacy is in doubt; their use results in little benefit to the patient and complicates an already crowded medication schedule. Questionable drugs are a significant cause of overmedication of the elderly and contribute to medication errors and drug reactions.

Dosage

When the dosage is in doubt, the lower amount in the range should be prescribed. Many very old patients who have been chronically ill weigh less than 90 pounds, and for them, the so-called geriatric dose may be quite excessive. A good rule for any prescriber treating the elderly is "go easy and go slow." Children who weigh more than 75 pounds can take an adult dose, but this shouldn't be applied to the elderly. Pediatric dosage is well worked out in comparison to geriatric dosage.

Directions to the patient should be clear and concise. "One or two tablets every three to four hours" may give the patient the idea that the schedule isn't critical or precise. He may then feel free to modify the directions in various ways (if one is good, two is better; three hours is better than four hours; and all through the night is better than just during the waking hours).

In regard to the quantity to be prescribed, it is better to err on the side of too little. Despite the large number of drugs ordered for older patients, the older patient has a relative intolerance to all kinds of medication. Drugs are expensive, and it's distressing, after prescribing a month's supply, to cancel the order after the second day. It's appropriate to order larger quantities of drugs only after one is certain of the patient's tolerance.

It's helpful to keep careful records of the amount of a drug prescribed, telephoned renewals, and the length of time the prescribed amount is expected to last. A request for premature renewal or delayed renewal may be the first warning of a medication problem. It also provides an opportunity to ask a family member to monitor drug usage in the interim between visits.

The patient should be encouraged to bring all his medications with him at each office visit. The physician should request the privilege of disposing of drugs not in current use and review the necessity of continuing all of the rest.

Dosage forms

Oral formulations are preferred. Liquids are better than solids, and granules are probably the least desirable. (We studied the use of granules and found that they have an affinity for the patient's dentures and also cause an inordinate water intake as the patient attempts to wash away all the granules out of the oral trap.) Small pills are better than large pills, and capsules are a happy medium. Splitting or crushing tablets is O.K. with some medications (see table with Chapter 6), but can be inaccurate.

Liquids offer the greatest flexibility, both in dosage and in mode of administration. If the patient's vision will not permit dosage measurement with a dropper, liquid concentrates can be diluted by the pharmacist to contain the desired amount in a teaspoonful. In addition, liquids can be mixed with a variety of fluids or foods for ease of administration.

Topical medications should be applied only in a thin film. Thick layers are wasteful and increase the chance that significant amounts will be absorbed. With potent preparations, this may result in a systemic effect when only a local one is intended. (I don't have experimental evidence for the possibility of increased drug absorption through the thin epidermis that is typical of the elderly, but it would seem likely.)

When more than one ophthalmic preparation is used in the same eye, the patient should be warned to allow at least several minutes between application of the drops, lest the second wash out the first before it has had time to exert an effect.

Suppositories requiring absorption of the active ingredients through the bowel wall will obviously be valueless when inserted into the center of a large fecal mass. The patient or whoever administers the drug should be told to make sure that the suppository lies against the mucosa.

SPECIFIC DRUG
CONSIDERATIONS

The following discussion focuses on specific aspects of drugs used in the treatment of the elderly.

Anabolic steroids and androgens

Use of these agents in the elderly is controversial. They're without value as a primary mode of treatment in senile or postmenopausal osteoporosis. They're contraindicated in carcinoma of the prostate or breast, and caution is advised for their use in the presence of cardiac, renal, or hepatic disease. There appears to be little reason for their use in geriatric medicine except for possibly the anemia of chronic renal disease and aplastic and hypoplastic anemia.

Analgesics

Aspirin is an effective analgesic but its use in the elderly is often excessive and unfortunately sometimes covert. Gastric irritation is a frequent side effect, and occult blood loss occurs in 50 to 70 per cent of the elderly who habitually take aspirin. In the presence of iron deficiency anemia, the patient and his family should be asked about the frequency and amount of aspirin use.

Acetaminophen is also an effective analgesic and produces less gastric irritation than aspirin. However, it doesn't have anti-inflammatory properties and so is not to be substituted when that effect is needed. In large doses, it may cause liver damage.

Phenylbutazone and indomethacin (Indocin) have both analgesic and anti-inflammatory properties, but may not be tolerated as well by the elderly as the two previously mentioned drugs. Ibuprofen (Motrin), tolmetin sodium (Tolectin), and naproxen (Naprosyn) are newer analgesics which are also anti-inflammatory agents and reportedly tend to have fewer side effects.

Although it's been clearly demonstrated that pain sensitivity decreases with age, pain is still one of the most common complaints of the elderly, and it requires skill in both diagnosis and management. Older patients in severe pain are too often given aspirin and other analgesics when, if the physician were the patient, he would be insisting on meperidine HCl (Demerol) to relieve the pain.

Fecal impactions are rather frequent in the elderly, and a narcotic should be given 20 to 30 minutes before digital removal of the impaction. When a narcotic is needed, a mild analgesic will not suffice. It's important, though, not to be in a hurry to relieve pain in the absence of a tenable diagnosis.

Antacids

Heartburn, epigastric distress, dyspepsia, and biliousness are reasons given by older people for the ingestion of such preparations as Rolaids, Alka-Seltzer, Pepto-Bismol, and a wide variety of aluminum hydroxide and/or magnesium trisilicate antacids. Excessive amounts of the latter drugs can cause diarrhea. The patient should be questioned about the use of aspirin, indomethacin, phenylbutazone, steroids, or chloral hydrate, because they may cause the distress.

Antianginal agents

Sublingual nitroglycerin is still the drug of choice for the acute attack of angina. In nursing homes, the attending physician must write an order that will permit the patient to have the medicine at the bedside. Unfortunately, many of these patients have difficulty in using sublingual medications properly. We've used a nitroglycerin ointment in some patients with gratifying results.

Propranolol HCl (Inderal) is very effective in preventing angina, but it may cause bradycardia, hypotension, hypoglycemia, and bronchospasm. It's therefore contraindicated in the presence of heart failure, heart block, or airway obstruction. Diabetic patients must be carefully observed since propranolol can mask the signs and symptoms of hypoglycemia.

Antibiotics

Antibiotics should be used with caution in the elderly. In this age group, ampicillin is one of the most common causes of skin rash. Ototoxic and nephrotoxic antibiotics, such as streptomycin sulfate, gentamicin (Garamycin), neomycin, and kanamycin, should be used cautiously. Tetracyclines accumulate in the body in the presence of altered renal function and can cause further renal damage, liver damage, and hyperuricemia. Lincomycin (Lincocin) and clindamycin

The King's Library

(Cleocin) are considered to be most likely to produce pseudomembranous colitis.

The question of when to treat urinary tract infections in the elderly has been debated. Many such infections that we've treated have often recurred. We've concluded that asymptomatic urinary tract infections in the elderly shouldn't be treated since (1) they almost inevitably recur unless a remediable condition is successfully treated and (2) they require the use of antibiotics that should be reserved for serious infections (indiscriminate use of antibiotics leads to an increase in resistant strains).

Anticoagulants

Older patients are very sensitive to anticoagulant therapy, and bleeding occurs twice as often as in the young. If prompt anticoagulation is needed, heparin is the drug of choice and should be given by continuous intravenous infusion after a loading dose. Warfarin is the preferred oral anticoagulant, but the initial dose should be about one-third that of a mature adult dose and the second dose should be delayed until after the prothrombin time is tested two days later.

Liver disease, phenylbutazone, salicylates, and broad-spectrum antibiotics can potentiate the action of warfarin. Discontinuance of certain drugs, such as phenobarbital, can have the same effect. Recent operations involving the eye or the central nervous system preclude the use of anticoagulants. Caution is advised in the presence of potential bleeding sites, as in ulcer disease, gastritis, and hiatal hernia accompanied by unexplained iron deficiency anemia.

Anticonvulsants

Seizure disorders are not uncommon in the elderly. Phenytoin, which may be used in this condition and also as an antiarrhythmic agent, may cause gingival hyperplasia, lymphadenopathy, and folate depletion resulting in megaloblastic anemia.

Antidepressants

The drugs most commonly used to treat depression are discussed in Chapter 3. We should note here, though, that drugs rank high as factors that precipitate depression. Among those most likely to be responsible are tranquilizers, sedatives, and antiemetics. Barbiturates may cause severe depression in a few patients; some of the phenothiazines, such as promazine and chlorpromazine, may also have this effect. Reserpine, which should rarely, if ever, be used in the elderly, can precipitate, aggravate, or prolong depression.

Antihypertensives

Both hypotension and hypertension are poorly tolerated in the elderly. Patients with diastolic blood pressures higher than 100 mm Hg and systolic pressures higher than 170 should generally be treated; however, these patients may tolerate therapy poorly, and therefore medication cannot be given to the point of effectiveness. A good rule of thumb is to start with the mildest regimen and modify it gradually as indicated. Weight reduction and salt restriction are rarely successful in the elderly unless stringently supervised. The next step is the introduction of thiazides with careful monitoring of the BUN and electrolytes, especially potassium, and avoidance of dehydration.

Reserpine should not be used because of the susceptibility of the elderly to drug-induced depression. Methyldopa may cause drowsiness and depression. About 20 per cent of the elderly patients receiving this drug develop a positive Coombs' test, but few progress to frank hemolytic anemia. Postural hypotension, however mild, is an indication to review the drugs being taken and to discontinue or decrease dosages.

Bronchodilators

Shortness of breath or wheezing may be due to cardiac as well as pulmonary problems. Oral xanthine preparations tend to cause nausea in the elderly and are better tolerated when administered by suppository or, in urgent circumstances, by intravenous drip. Patients older than age 75 don't manage sprays or inhalants very well, especially when administration and inhalation must be coordinated.

Cerebral vasodilators

There has been much interest in whether the supply of blood to the brain can be increased in the elderly by cerebral vasodilators and whether clinical improvement ensues and can be maintained. We'd welcome definite evidence that this approach can delay or decelerate mental deterioration. Because we have little else to offer, these drugs can be given for several weeks to one month, after which their continued use can be considered.

Corticosteroids

Corticosteroids should be used with considerable caution in the elderly since there's increased danger of accelerating osteoporosis, precipitating peptic ulceration, and promoting fluid retention. These agents can also cause stable diabetes to go out of control and can change a manageable patient into one with behavior problems.

Cough preparations

Cough suppressants shouldn't be used unless the cough is due to malignancy and is very distressing to the patient. A codeine preparation may be given but may cause constipation. If this isn't efficacious, it may be necessary to use methadone. There are many cough preparations that help loosen secretions, and the patient expects some type of medication regardless of its effectiveness. Use of a vaporizer or heated aerosol will provide considerable relief.

Digitalis

Early signs of digitalis toxicity in the elderly are drowsiness, fatigue, and confusion. The main difference in digoxin metabolism in the elderly is the substantial reduction in the rate of renal excretion. The loading dose in older patients is one-half that for younger patients (0.5 to 0.75 mg as compared to 1.0 to 1.5 mg), and the usual maintenance dose is now 0.125 mg daily. In older people, especially those with renal impairment, careful observation is essential since serum digoxin levels don't always correlate closely with clinical and electrocardiographic evidence of toxicity. Geriatric patients are particularly prone to adverse effects that are frequently atypical.

Diuretics

Older people who feel ill will frequently stop food and fluid intake. One or two days of self-imposed fasting can result in dehydration and electrolyte imbalance. If the person is taking digitalis the problem is compounded, and if he is also on diuretics, management of all factors is essential for the patient's recovery. If thiazides are used, potassium supplementation may be necessary. However, if the patient is taking a potassium-sparing diuretic in conjunction with a thiazide, potassium supplementation shouldn't be used. The most common cause of edema in the elderly (in the absence of congestive heart failure) is venous stasis, which shouldn't be treated with diuretics.

Hematinics

Accurate diagnosis is critical for the proper management of anemia. In a case of iron deficiency anemia, failure to respond to iron therapy within a three-month period is indicative of either a wrong diagnosis or an overlooked or occult lesion. A blood transfusion should never be given to a moderately to severely anemic patient without a thorough investigation. The blood is merely a stopgap measure that may not only be dangerous in its own right but may also mask pernicious anemia or delay the diagnosis of a lesion beyond the point at which it can successfully be treated.

Malnutrition is fairly common in older people and increases the risk of nutritional anemias, including folate deficiency. If vitamin B_{12} deficiency is present or coexists with folate deficiency, and the problem is treated solely with folic acid, there is danger of later subacute combined degeneration of the spinal cord. It may be advisable to administer vitamin B_{12} to all patients receiving folate. If the nutritional problems can't be corrected, folate may have to be given indefinitely.

Unfortunately, some anemic patients defy diagnosis and don't respond to therapy. Success in diagnosis may be commensurate with the insight and effort that are applied to the problem.

Hypoglycemics

Diabetes therapy poses special problems in the elderly. When possible, weight loss and observation of dietary restrictions are helpful in the control of diabetes. However, adherence to a strict diet can't be relied on; it's a delusion of those who care for their parents and grandparents. Cheating is so common that the use of a strict diabetic diet must be discounted.

Among the oral antidiabetes agents, the two main drugs currently used are tolbutamide and chlorpropamide (Diabinese). Because chlorpropamide has a 36-hour half-life, it tends to be cumulative if given daily, and the effects of overdosage are slow to appear and disappear. Despite this disadvantage, it's probably the better initial drug for the elderly since tolbutamide action lasts about eight hours and therefore may have to be given more than once daily for optimal control.

Insulin injections are difficult for elderly patients to administer, mainly because of failing vision, confusion, and loss of manual dexterity. Many older diabetics must rely on someone else for proper administration of insulin.

Sedatives and hypnotics

Barbiturates should not be used as sedatives or hypnotics because they frequently cause confusion and, if sleep is interrupted for a trip to the bathroom, the result may be a fall with significant injury. Tranquilizers are better sedatives. Chloral hydrate, flurazepam HCl (Dalmane) in one-half the usual adult dose, or, when indicated, a tricyclic antidepressant given as a single bedtime dose can be successfully used as a hypnotic.

Tranquilizers

While tranquilizers don't cloud consciousness as much as the barbiturates, they do tend to produce postural hypotension, which can result in accidental injuries. The major tranquilizers may cause signs and symptoms of parkinsonism, especially weakness, restlessness, uncoordinated movements, tremors, and rigidity. Antiparkinsonian drugs are often administered with the major tranquilizers in the hope of avoiding extrapyramidal side effects; however, these agents may decrease the effectiveness of the tranquilizer without affecting the incidence of side effects, including tardive dyskinesia. It's of utmost importance that a thorough examination and documentation be made before starting patients on antiparkinsonian medications.

The presence of extrapyramidal motion disturbances, skin eruptions, electrocardiographic changes, and ocular opacities should be specifically noted. It's important to realize that failure to record the absence of each of these conditions may be construed as evidence that they were not present rather than that they were not specifically looked for.

Case reports of sudden, unexpected death in patients taking large amounts of neuroleptics have appeared in the literature. A major concern is the rapidly rising incidence of tardive dyskinesia since the advent of the major tranquilizers. We're dealing with very potent agents whose end targets are the binding sites in the nervous system and whose effects, once entrenched, aren't reversible. It behooves us, perhaps, to use a smaller stick or to wield the large one we have with a little less force.

Vitamins

For many medical, social, and economic reasons, nutritional problems abound in the elderly. We have already mentioned the use of vitamin B_{12} and folic acid in the treatment of anemia. If the nutritional status and the nutritional history of the patient indicate malnutrition, the patient should be given a vitamin-mineral supplement. A therapeutic formula may be used initially, but after several days to one week, the patient should be given a maintenance formula.

The pluses and minuses of eight drug administration routes

Oral. This is the oldest, safest, most convenient, and most economical route. The disadvantages are possible emesis resulting from irritation of the gastrointestinal mucosa, destruction of the drug by digestive enzymes, binding of the drug with food into unabsorbable complexes, and the necessity for cooperation from the patient.

Sublingual. Absorption from oral mucosa is rapid. It permits a higher concentration in the blood because the drug doesn't have to go through the liver where it can be metabolically reduced. However, irritating or bad-tasting drugs can't be given this way.

Rectal. This is useful if the patient is vomiting or unconscious, and the drug doesn't have to pass through the liver. Absorption, however, is often irregular or incomplete, and the drug may irritate the mucosa.

Intramuscular. Drugs in aqueous solution injected deep into muscle are absorbed rapidly and predictably. Parenteral administration is especially useful in emergency therapy or if the patient is unconscious, uncooperative, or unable to retain anything given by mouth. Disadvantages include the need for strict asepsis, limited opportunity for the patient to medicate himself, and expense.

Intravenous. The desired blood concentration and precise amount are obtained with an immediacy no other route can give. It provides the only route for certain irritating and hypertonic solutions. The danger from infection is high, repeated injections depend on patency of veins, and the form is expensive.

Subcutaneous. The rate of absorption is often sufficiently slow and even to provide a sustained effect. But irritating drugs can make affected tissue slough. Like other parenteral routes, it's more expensive and inconvenient.

Inhalation. Gaseous and volatile drugs may be delivered directly to the sites where needed in certain pulmonary diseases without the delay and possible adverse effects of a systemic route. Absorption by the circulation is almost instantaneous.

Mucous membranes. Absorption is fairly rapid through mucous membranes of the oropharynx, nose, conjunctiva, urethra, and vagina. Irritating drugs can't be given this way.

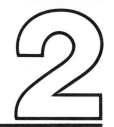

How Aging Alters the Actions of Drugs

By Zachary I. Hanan, R.Ph., M.S.

As your patients grow old, they suffer more diseases, often several at the same time. They seek care not only in geriatric services and nursing homes, but also in medical and surgical units of acute-care hospitals, outpatient departments, clinics, and doctors' offices. So unless you work exclusively with children, you'll likely find yourself increasingly responsible for the care of aging patients.

Because they're ill so often, people older than 65 are frequently subject to adverse reactions and to drug interactions from taking several medications at the same time. Ironically, their drug-induced illnesses may escape detection because the symptoms often mimic the stereotyped characteristics of old age: forgetfulness, weakness, confusion, tremor, anorexia, and anxiety.

But that's just the beginning of the problems you'll encounter in drug therapy for the aged. In addition, the elderly undergo physiological changes independent of any disease state, a number of the changes occurring at the cellular level. Parenchymal cells (the functional cells of an organ) show a reduction in number and a decrease in the rate of turnover. The heart, brain, kidney, lungs, and muscle can suffer as much as 40 per cent loss of cell population by the age of 75. Nondividing cells such as those in the nervous system also show a progressive reduction in numbers.

Thus, let us say that if an organ has lost 30 per cent of its cells, the 70 per cent remaining may function adequately under normal physiological conditions. But what happens under stress? The organ is 30 per cent deficient in meeting body needs, a point not to be overlooked in drug therapy.

It is necessary to remember that a drug introduced into the body may act as a stress or stress-inducer, and, additionally, that side effects of drugs can be considered stresses—all more difficult for the elderly patient than the younger patient to overcome.

Also, these changes in body structure and functioning can weaken, strengthen, or significantly alter a drug's action. They affect the ways that drugs are absorbed, distributed throughout the body, metabolized, and excreted.

Absorption

Because the stomach is normally quite acidic, orally administered acidic drugs—for example, aspirin—are rapidly absorbed into the bloodstream. But in old people, the pH of the stomach is higher (less acid), and this is likely to slow the absorption of acidic drugs. A consistently higher pH may also explain why serum levels of vitamin B_{12} are lower in the old. You can expect elderly patients to absorb drugs erratically and slowly. However, the total amount will usually be absorbed.

Distribution

After absorption into the bloodstream, many drugs are stored in various parts of the body, including fat and serum protein. The drugs are then returned to the blood as needed in order to keep the concentration in equilibrium.

Physiology of the elderly

Organ or organ system	Changes and results	Effects on drug use
Immune system	Responds more slowly and less vigorously to invading bacteria/viruses, producing greater susceptibility to infections	Increased use of antibiotics and cough/cold preparations
Cardiovascular	Due to arterio-atherosclerosis, vital heart-function decrease (1 per cent per year after body reaches full maturity); gradual increase in blood pressure; congestive heart failure	Increased use of digitalis preparations and antihypertensive agents
Kidney	Decreased function as patient ages: 65 years old, 30 per cent decrease 90 years old, 50 per cent decrease	Increased chance of toxicity with the use of drugs cleared by the kidney
Gastrointestinal	Erratic and slow absorption of drugs; constipation	Unexpected or prolonged effect of drugs; chronic use of laxatives
Hematological	Anemia (usually not iron)	Especially during certain drug regimens, the following supplements may be needed: folic acid, cyanocobalamin, iron

Organ or organ system	Changes and results	Effects on drug use
Pulmonary	Loss of functional units of the lung, worsening other diseases; congestive heart failure; emphysema	Increased administration of drugs used in obstructive lung disease
Genitourinary	Increase in infections and/or urinary retention	Treatment required for urinary tract infections and prostatitis
Musculoskeletal	Osteoporosis, osteoarthritis, and rheumatoid arthritis	Increased use of anti-inflammatory agents
Hormonal	Females—menopause; males—decrease in testosterone; greater incidence of diabetes	Estrogen added to female drug regimen, no specific drug used for males; more use of insulin and oral hypoglycemics
CNS	Athero- and arteriosclerotic changes; changes in sleep patterns, with early awakening common	Greater sensitivity to hypnotic effects of drugs, causing CNS signs; increased use of and sensitivity to CNS depressants
Hepatic	Metabolic slowdown (not documented in man); extreme sensitivity to lack of oxygen, secondary to heart failure, anemia, hardening of arteries—all of which may compromise function	Affects, theoretically, any drug metabolized in the liver

In aging persons, the proportion of total body fluid and lean body mass decreases, and much of the metabolically active tissue is replaced by fat. Some drugs—for example, phenobarbital, diazepam (Valium), and chlorpromazine—are fat soluble. If you give an elderly patient a weight-related dose of a fat-soluble drug, more of it will go into storage. As a result, you'll see a decreased intensity of effect, but a prolonged duration of action. Given over a long period, a fat-soluble drug can accumulate in the body and produce toxic effects.

Many drugs become bound to serum proteins, especially to albumin. If the affinity is high, the albumin may serve as the reservoir and release the drug into the blood as it's needed. Serum albumin levels are lower in elderly patients, but the effect of this lower level on the action of protein-bound drugs has never been fully investigated. There is some evidence that protein binding of phenytoin and warfarin (Coumadin, Panwarfin) is less, so the drugs are more immediately available. No change has been seen in the protein binding of phenobarbital, penicillin G, diazepam, salicylate, and sulfadiazine (Suladyne).

Other characteristics of old age may also alter distribution. Starting at age 19, cardiac output decreases. The demands of the heart and brain to be the first supplied from a decreasing output may lead to an accumulation of drugs in those organs.

There's also speculation that the penetration of some CNS drugs into spinal fluid changes with old age. Are, for example, the increased analgesic effects of morphine and pentazocine (Talwin) related to increased penetration? May that also explain the elderly's experiencing increased ototoxicity from aminoglycoside antibiotics such as kanamycin sulfate (Kantrex) and streptomycin sulfate?

Metabolism

All ingested drugs eventually pass through the liver. Some emerge unchanged, but most undergo a metabolic detoxification process in which liver microsomal enzymes break the drugs down into water-soluble substances for excretion by the kidneys. The duration of action and intensity of effect of many drugs depends largely on the number of microsomal enzymes and the speed at which they work. Many drugs, including phenobarbital, stimulate the liver to synthesize increased amounts of enzymes. This process is called enzyme induction. If you give phenobarbital and warfarin together, the anti-

How orally administered drugs get into the bloodstream

A molecule of a drug generally consists of a positively charged part and a negatively charged part. If the positively charged part and negatively charged part of all the molecules start drifting away from each other as the drug goes into solution in the stomach, the drug is said to be ionized. But if the two charged parts of each molecule stay together, the drug is non-ionized. Ionized drugs aren't lipid soluble. Non-ionized drugs are. This distinction is crucial because of what happens next.

Between the internal mucosal lining of the gastrointestinal tract and the bloodstream is a microscopically thin layer of tissue called the lipoidal layer. This layer is selectively permeable: It bars the passage of non-lipid-soluble substances (ionized drugs) into the bloodstream, but permits the passage of lipid-soluble substances (non-ionized drugs).

Most drugs are weak acids or weak bases. The high acidity of the stomach keeps the weakly acidic drugs non-ionized, so they are rapidly absorbed. The weakly basic drugs remain ionized in the stomach and so resist absorption. But as they move from the stomach to the small intestines, they encounter a change in pH from acidity to alkalinity. The weakly basic drugs go from their ionized state to a non-ionized state and are absorbed. Drugs and other substances that are strongly acidic or strongly basic remain ionized throughout and are poorly absorbed in both the stomach and the small intestine.

Some examples of weakly acidic drugs are barbiturates, coumarin, urinary germicides (nalidixic acid, methenamine, and nitrofurantoin), phenylbutazone, and sulfonamides.

Some examples of weakly basic drugs are amphetamine, narcotic analgesics (morphine, codeine, and meperidine), antiarrhythmics (quinidine and procainamide), tricyclic antidepressants (amitriptyline, imipramine, and desipramine), and sympathomimetic drugs (ephedrine, epinephrine, and isoproterenol).

coagulant is more quickly metabolized, and its therapeutic effect diminished. The metabolism of phenobarbital itself is rapid.

The liver's capacity to metabolize drugs decreases with age. One reason may be that an inadequate intake of protein reduces the amount of metabolizing enzymes. Whatever the reason, the result is that unmetabolized drugs continue to exert their effects. Particularly with drugs that are quickly deactivated by the liver in younger patients—for example, meperidine HCl (Demerol), barbiturates, propranolol HCl (Inderal), and tricyclic antidepressants—you may see prolonged effects in the elderly. On the other hand, with a drug that needs to be metabolized for full therapeutic effect, such as allopurinol (Zyloprim), you may observe reduced effectiveness.

Excretion

For most drugs, the kidneys are the main route of elimination. For some, especially many antibiotics and some cardiac glycosides, they are virtually the only route. Three processes are involved: passive glomerular filtration, active tubular secretion and reabsorption, and passive tubular diffusion.

Dehydration in elderly patients

Ann Boylan, R.N., M.A., and Bernard Marbach, M.D.

Dehydration is one of the most common geriatric problems, plaguing nursing home and hospital patients alike. Untreated, it can quickly lead to severe electrolyte imbalance, shock, renal failure, coma, convulsions, and death. Even in its early stages, it places an added strain on body systems already debilitated by age and illness, contributing to such problems as recurrent urinary tract infection, skin breakdown, and constipation.

All elderly patients are at some risk of dehydration, but some are more vulnerable than others. These vulnerable patients should be identified and closely monitored for deviations in food and fluid intake and for signs of dehydration.

The best way to prevent dehydration or arrest it at an early stage is, of course, to encourage fluid intake at every opportunity. However, even the best efforts at preventing dehydration may not always work. If a patient won't or can't take sufficient fluids by mouth, water and electrolyte deficits must be remedied by some other means and without delay. The two major treatment methods are parenteral administration of fluids by either the intravenous or subcutaneous route, and tube feeding. See the August 1979 issue of *RN* magazine for ways to prevent dehydration and for more details concerning its treatment.

One of the tables presented here explains why the elderly become dehydrated. Another lists the patients who are most likely to suffer dehydration, and the third gives early signs that suggest dehydration may have already set in.

Dehydration in elderly patients (continued)

Why the elderly become dehydrated

Intake			Output		
Water and other beverages	1200 ml		Insensible water loss	Lungs	700 ml
Water from food	1100 ml			Skin	300 ml
Water of oxidation (12 cc/100 cal)	300 ml		Observable water loss	Sweat	100 ml
				Feces	100 ml
				Urine	1400 ml
Total	**2600 ml**		**Total**		**2600 ml**

Generally, the human body has no difficulty maintaining water balance. This chart shows the average normal bodily exchange of water in a temperate climate.* But the debilities that often accompany advancing age can conspire to upset this balance.

Many elderly people simply don't take in enough food and/or water to maintain adequate fluid levels, because of such factors as deteriorating mental function, depression and loss of interest, difficulty in feeding themselves, and illness and general debilitation. Nor do they respond to the physical signals of water loss.

Normally, a person consumes fluids in response to thirst. The thirst center in the hypothalamus is activated by hyperosmolar imbalance—excessive amounts of sodium in relation to water in body fluids. When the body either loses water or gains sodium, the osmolarity (number of dissolved particles per liter) of the extracellular

*Modified and reproduced with permission from Hoffman WS: *The Biochemistry of Clinical Medicine* (4th ed). Copyright © 1970 by Year Book Medical Publishers Inc., Chicago

Dehydration in elderly patients
Why the elderly become dehydrated (continued)

fluid increases, causing water from inside the cells to shift into the extracellular fluid to restore balance. The resulting drop in intracellular fluid levels stimulates receptors in the hypothalamus, which transmits impulses to the cerebral cortex and brings about a desire to drink.

However, recognizing and responding to thirst is a conscious act and therefore inoperative in unconscious, semiconscious, confused, or even severely depressed patients—categories into which many of the elderly fall. (To complicate the situation, many conditions—for example, hemorrhage, severe vomiting, and diarrhea—may cause loss of large amounts of both water and sodium in roughly equal proportions. When this happens, fluid volume is depleted but no imbalance occurs to activate the thirst center, so the patient may not experience thirst at all.)

When the body doesn't take in enough water to allow for excretion of wastes by the kidneys, it begins to draw on fluid reserves in the tissues. Fluid reserves tend to decrease with age, leaving the elderly more vulnerable to dehydration when inadequate intake forces the body to draw on these reserves.

Urine output is the most controllable component of water loss, and healthy kidneys with normal circulation and normal fluid reserves to draw upon can usually maintain a fine water balance. However, both circulation and kidney function are often compromised in the elderly, leaving the kidneys with diminished ability to concentrate urine and hence a precarious control over urine output. Disruption of the water balance and dehydration further compromise kidney circulation and function, and compound the problem in a vicious cycle.

Dehydration in elderly patients (continued)

Patients vulnerable to dehydration

- Patients who are unconscious, semiconscious, confused, or severely depressed.

- Patients on tube feedings or intravenous infusion.

- Patients who have to be fed or require help feeding themselves because of visual impairment, paralysis, severe arthritis, or some other problem.

- Patients with poor appetites.

- Patients who are chair- or bedbound.

- Patients on large doses of tranquilizers or sedatives.

- Patients on diuretics such as furosemide (Lasix), ethacrynic acid (Edecrin), or the thiazides (hydrochlorothiazide, for example).

- Patients who use laxatives frequently or have frequent enemas.

- Patients who have suffered fluid losses because of hemorrhage, vomiting, diarrhea, excessive urination, diaphoresis, hyperventilation (leading to excessive water loss through the lungs), or excessive sputum production.

Dehydration in elderly patients (continued)
Dehydration checklist

Keep in mind the following questions when you are assessing elderly patients for early signs of dehydration. The more "yes" answers you come up with, the more suspicious you should be—and the more attentive to the patient's fluid needs.

● Does the patient complain of thirst?

● Are his lips and/or conjunctiva dry? Are his mucosa sticky?

● Is his tongue swollen?

● Are his eyeballs sunken? Does he have dark circles underneath his eyes?

● Is his temperature above normal?

● Is his blood pressure below normal?

● Is his urine output lower and more concentrated than usual?

● Is he constipated?

● Is he losing weight?

● Does he seem unusually agitated or disoriented?

● Is he nauseated or vomiting?

● Has he recently experienced diarrhea? Excessive urination (such as that associated with uncontrolled diabetes mellitus)? Diaphoresis?

● Is he hyperventilating?

● Is he producing large amounts of sputum?

● Has his food and fluid intake decreased?

● Do lab studies, if available, show: Elevated hematocrit? Elevated hemoglobin? Urine specific gravity above 1.030? Elevated BUN, serum sodium, or serum protein? Decreased urine chloride (below 50 mEq/l)?

All these processes lose their efficiency in old age. In a person of 65, the glomerular filtration rate is about 30 per cent slower than that in a young adult. Tubular secretion also deteriorates. Penicillin, one of several drugs that are eliminated by tubular secretion, saturates the failing tubules in elderly patients and thus remains active in the bloodstream.

Impairment of renal function combined with decreased ability of the liver to detoxify plus a higher proportion of body weight turning to drug-storing fat can cause even moderate dosages of drugs to accumulate quickly to toxic levels. In addition, an aging patient is also susceptible to renal impairment caused by dehydration, congestive heart failure, hypotension, and urinary retention resulting from diseases such as diabetic nephropathy and pyelonephritis.

Many aging persons whose health and reserves are only marginal are nevertheless functioning and independent. But an unwanted drug response can push them over the brink into confusion, incompetence, and helplessness. It's our obligation as health-care professionals to carry out their drug therapy with more than usual care.

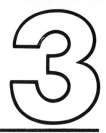

How Psychotropic Drugs Can Go Astray

By Marc Bachinsky, R.Ph., M.S.

Advancing age often produces a complex interaction of physical and mental illness and decreased capacity to perceive, analyze, and remember. With some older people, it takes longer for new data to sink in, and they appear to have memory defects. Depression can compound the problem.

There are many factors that bring on depression in the elderly. Many in retirement feel useless; without income, they worry about finances, and sometimes a lower income brings on lower self-esteem. Becoming the victim of a disease that is thought to be typical of old age can be a cause of depression. Too, the death of one's spouse or friend is an obvious loss that can put the elderly survivor into a depressed state.

Though depression is common, it can easily be missed—most often, by attributing its symptoms to senility. Depression in patients with arteriosclerosis and borderline senility accentuates the symptoms of the physiological disorder. If the depression is treated, the patient may recover well enough from it to compensate for the physiological disorder. Since depression is treatable, it pays to be on the lookout for it and to deal with it.

Drug therapy is essential for managing depression, whatever its origin, but it's tricky to use because the aging process often interferes with the expected effects. Moreover, the use of psychotropic drugs may severely complicate treatment of cardiovascular disorders, respiratory problems, liver or renal dysfunctions, cancer, diabetes, or malnutrition—all of which occur frequently among the elderly. The physician should give a careful physical examination and treat the medical condition first.

Once the physician decides to proceed with a psychotropic drug, he can follow guidelines to the safest possible use of these drugs in the elderly. These guidelines include:

• making an accurate diagnosis unswayed by inexact impressions offered by the patient's family;

- keeping the number of drugs prescribed to a minimum;
- starting therapy with small doses and increasing them only gradually;
- ordering periodic lab tests, such as blood counts, to monitor cumulative toxicity; and
- avoiding a premature switch to another drug because there's no immediate response.

Adverse reactions

Unfavorable reactions affect almost all body systems in elderly patients, but some more seriously than others. In the cardiovascular system, antipsychotic and tricyclic antidepressants can produce severe orthostatic hypotension and syncope. High doses of minor tranquilizers can cause hypotensive episodes, and MAO inhibitors can produce either hypotensive or hypertensive reactions. Phenothiazines and tricyclic antidepressants have been implicated in congestive heart failure, massive edema, and sudden death.

Gastrointestinal reactions are less of a problem because most oral psychotropic drugs are readily absorbed, even in the elderly.

Guide to adverse effects of psychotropic drugs in the elderly

The adverse effects identified here may occur in patients of all ages, but the frequency is much higher and complications usually more serious in elderly patients.

Drug	Condition treated	Possible adverse effects
Antihistamines Diphenhydramine HCl	Insomnia, sleep disorders	Confusion, nervousness, restlessness, nausea, vomiting, diarrhea, blurred vision, urinary retention, hypotension, dry mouth
Barbiturates Amobarbital Butabarbital Pentobarbital (Nembutal) Phenobarbital Secobarbital	Insomnia, sleep disorders	Respiratory depression, circulatory collapse, skin rash, lethargy, headache, nausea, vomiting, decrease in potency of coumarin anticoagulants, prolonged effect (from short- and intermediate-acting barbiturates) in patients with impaired hepatic function

Benzodiazepines
Chlordiazepoxide
Clorazepate
  (Tranxene)
Diazepam
  (Valium)
	Anxiety	Drowsiness, ataxia, confusion, dizziness, dry mouth, blurred vision, headache, fatigue, constipation, hypotension, urinary retention

Drug	Condition treated	Possible adverse effects
Benzodiazepines Lorazepam (Ativan) Oxazepam (Serax) Prazepam (Verstran)	Anxiety	Drowsiness, ataxia, confusion, dizziness, dry mouth, blurred vision, headache, fatigue, constipation, hypotension, urinary retention
Butyrophenones Haloperidol (Haldol)	Psychotic disorders	Extrapyramidal reactions similar to parkinsonism, tardive dyskinesia (especially in old women), insomnia, anxiety, restlessness, tachycardia, hypotension, anorexia, constipation, nausea, vomiting, blurred vision, urinary retention
Chloral derivatives Chloral betaine Chloral hydrate Triclofos sodium (Triclos)	Insomnia, sleep disorders	Moderate gastrointestinal upset, cumulative toxicity in patients with marked renal or hepatic impairment
Dibenzoxazepines Loxapine (Daxolin, Loxitane)	Schizophrenia	Extrapyramidal reactions similar to parkinsonism, tardive dyskinesia (especially in old women), tachycardia, hypotension, dermatitis, edema

Guide to adverse effects of
psychotropic drugs in the elderly (continued)

Drug	Condition treated	Possible adverse effects
Dihydroindolones Molindone (Lidone, Moban)	Schizophrenia	Initial drowsiness, extrapyramidal reactions, blurred vision, tachycardia, nausea, dry mouth, urinary retention, tardive dyskinesia
MAO inhibitors Phenelzine (Nardil) Tranylcypromine (Parnate)	Depression	Dizziness, constipation, dry mouth, postural hypotension, weakness, fatigue, edema, serious and possibly fatal hypertensive crisis when given with sympathomimetic drugs or aged cheese, beer, wine, pickled herring, and chicken liver
Phenothiazines Chlorpromazine Fluphenazine HCl (Prolixin, Permitil) Mesoridazine (Serentil) Perphenazine Piperacetazine (Quide) Prochlorperazine Thioridazine (Mellaril) Trifluoperazine HCl (Stelazine) Triflupromazine (Vesprin)	Psychotic disorders	Extrapyramidal reactions similar to parkinsonism, tardive dyskinesia, hypotension, blood dyscrasias, itching, urinary retention

Drug	Condition treated	Possible adverse effects
Piperidine derivatives Glutethimide Methyprylon (Noludar)	Insomnia, sleep disorders	Morning drowsiness, dizziness, diarrhea, nausea, vomiting, headache
Stimulants Dextroamphetamine Methamphetamine HCl (Desoxyn) Methylphenidate HCl (Ritalin)	Depression	Palpitation, tachycardia, hypertension, restlessness, insomnia, tremor, headache, dry mouth, diarrhea, constipation
Thioxanthenes Chlorprothixene (Taractan) Thiothixene (Navane)	Psychotic disorders	Extrapyramidal reactions similar to parkinsonism, tardive dyskinesia, hypotension, blood dyscrasias, itching, urinary retention
Tricyclic derivatives Amitriptyline HCl (Elavil)	Depression	Hypotension, hypertension, tachycardia, myocardial infarction, arrhythmias, confusion, anxiety, restlessness, extrapyramidal reactions, dry mouth,

Guide to adverse effects of
psychotropic drugs in the elderly (continued)

Drug	Condition treated	Possible adverse effects
Tricyclic derivatives Desipramine HCl (Norpramin, Pertofrane) Doxepin (Sinequan) Imipramine HCl Nortriptyline HCl (Aventyl, Pamelor) Protriptyline HCl (Vivactil)	Depression	blurred vision, increased intraocular pressure, paralytic ileus, urinary retention, skin rash, edema, nausea, vomiting

The most serious reactions are paralytic ileus and toxic megacolon. These effects are related to cholinergic blocking action, to which the elderly are especially susceptible.

Extrapyramidal reactions—neuromuscular activity involving postural, static, and locomotor mechanisms—are a common neurological problem in elderly patients taking psychotropic drugs. Antiparkinsonism agents like benztropine mesylate (Cogentin) control the symptoms well, but they add to the anticholinergic effects of antipsychotic and antidepressant drugs. For this reason, it's better to reduce the dosage of the drug that causes the problem than to treat the problem with another drug.

Tardive dyskinesia, to which elderly women taking antipsychotic drugs are especially susceptible, doesn't respond well to antiparkinsonism drugs. Other central nervous system reactions to psychotropic drugs that are especially severe or common among the elderly are depression, paradoxical agitation, delirium, confusion, assaultiveness, delusions, and hallucination.

Antipsychotic, antidepressant, and antiparkinsonism drugs block cholinergic action, which can be dangerous for elderly patients with disturbed cardiac rhythm. Cholinergic blockade can also produce dry mouth, loss of ocular accommodation, constipation, hypotension, loss of coordination, vertigo, sweating, urinary retention, atonic bladder, and increased intraocular pressure.

Elderly patients also run a greater risk of suffering allergic reactions to psychotropic drugs. Among these reactions are blood dyscrasias—chiefly agranulocytosis and thrombocytopenia—cholestatic jaundice, dermatitis, photosensitivity, pigmentary changes, and eye damage.

Major tranquilizers

Aliphatic phenothiazines—for example, chlorpromazine—are highly sedative and have a marked tendency to cause hypotension. This limits their usefulness in elderly patients who sleep during the day instead of at night or who have cardiovascular disease. Haloperidol (Haldol) and piperazine phenothiazines, such as trifluoperazine HCl (Stelazine), produce little sedation and hypotension, but are more likely to cause extrapyramidal reactions. Nevertheless, the low incidence of cardiovascular side effects seen with haloperidol make it a good agent in patients who have blood pressure problems.

Manic behavior occurs less frequently in elderly patients than it does in younger adults. When it does occur, lithium carbonate is the drug of choice. You have to monitor elderly patients on lithium closely for cardiovascular, thyroid, and renal function to avoid toxicity. The usual starting dose for an elderly patient is 300 mg two to three times daily until the blood level is 1.2 mEq/l. The recommended maintenance dose is 300 mg daily.

Depression

Not surprisingly, depression is the most common psychiatric disorder among the elderly. Tricyclic antidepressants are effective, but their onset of action may be delayed as long as three weeks after therapy begins. Elderly patients should be started on doses no higher than 40 mg daily and increased no faster than 25 mg per week to a maximum of 150 mg daily.

Elderly patients are more likely to suffer from *agitated* depression than from *retarded* depression. In agitated depression, antidepressants with sedative action, such as doxepin HCl (Adapin, Sinequan) and amitriptyline HCl, may be more helpful than anti-

Problems of simple aging

Problems	Causes	Management
Social	Abandonment by family Decreased mobility Fear of losing economic security Lack of social interaction Loss of ability to attain goals Loss of occupational interests and productivity Loss of role identity Reduced income	Family involvement Economic counseling or financial assistance Social interaction Avocational interests Stimulation of self-esteem through exercise, decision-making, responsibility, good appearance Part-time jobs Improved housing
Psychological	Decreased influence over environment Fear of aloneness Fear of death Loss of loved ones	Environmental manipulation Psychotherapeutic counseling Psychotropic medication
Physiological	Brain-tissue changes Decreasing motor strength Sensory losses (hearing, smell, taste, and vision)	Improvement of brain function with medication Correction of sensory deficits (refraction, cataract surgery, hearing aids) Diagnosis and treatment of underlying physical disorders Physical rehabilitation

depressants with stimulant properties, such as protriptyline HCl (Vivactil), desipramine HCl (Norpramin, Pertofrane), tranylcypromine sulfate (Parnate), phenelzine sulfate (Nardil), and nortriptyline HCl (Aventyl, Pamelor).

If your geriatric patient has urinary incontinence, you may help him by capitalizing on the side effects of imipramine HCl and certain other tricyclic antidepressants. These drugs, which produce urinary retention and delayed micturition in patients with normal urinary function, can help incontinent patients achieve control within a few days at a dosage of 10 to 25 mg t.i.d. This effect is probably unrelated to the drugs' mood-lifting properties.

Tricyclic antidepressants are usually quite safe for physically healthy young adults; the most common side effects are transient drowsiness, dry mouth, and blurred vision. In the elderly, they can cause confusion, more serious problems like agranulocytosis and paralytic ileus, and even fatal heart disorders. Response to tricyclic antidepressants varies widely, so a medication history is the best guide to selecting a drug.

MAO inhibitors aren't used routinely in the elderly because of their toxic interactions with many drugs and foods. Psychomotor

Recognizing causes of aberrant behavior

How a patient acts	What it can mean	How a patient acts	What it can mean
Cries periodically. States he wishes to die. States he feels hopeless. Doesn't care for personal appearance. Doesn't eat. Can't sleep.	Depression	Can't give name. Doesn't know the time or place. Can't recognize familiar people.	Disorientation
Refuses to leave his room. Refuses to eat or sit with other patients. Doesn't talk to anyone.	Withdrawal	Climbs into another patient's bed. Removes clothes. Extinguishes cigarettes on table. Wanders aimlessly. Urinates in room.	Confusion
Paces in halls. Constantly wrings hands. Picks at bedclothes and self. Constantly moves about when sitting.	Agitation	States someone is in the closet or under the bed. Refuses to eat or take medications, saying someone is trying to kill him. States a fixed but unrealistic belief.	Delusions
Talks to "someone" who is not there. Hears or sees an invisible person or object.	Hallucination	Threatens to hurt other patients. Strikes out at staff. Demands constant attention. Shouts at staff and patients.	Aggression

stimulants aren't useful for treating depression in the elderly because they often cause agitation, confusion, and disorientation. In low doses, however, they may benefit apathetic elderly patients.

Barbiturates were once widely used as antianxiety agents, but they've been largely replaced by other less toxic drugs. Nevertheless, habituation to these drugs remains a problem, and abrupt withdrawal can cause delirium and seizures. Benzodiazepine drugs, which include chlordiazepoxide and diazepam (Valium), are the safest and most effective antianxiety agents.

Organic brain syndrome

At least 50 per cent of elderly patients in mental hospitals and nursing homes and 30 per cent of other elderly patients suffer from organic brain syndromes. In acute syndromes, the underlying cause can usually be identified and controlled. Until it's controlled, the patient may show symptoms of agitation and assaultiveness, but he may respond to an antipsychotic agent such as a phenothiazine drug.

In chronic organic brain syndrome, a vasodilating drug like papaverine may help by increasing blood flow to ischemic areas of the brain. Patient improvement is evident in socializing and behavior, but not in intellectual functioning. Hydergine, a dehydrogenated ergot alkaloid that modifies brain-cell metabolism, can produce a similar improvement.

Hypnotics

Many elderly patients have difficulty falling asleep or they wake too early. Early waking may be a sign of depression; if it's overcome by an antidepressant and psychotherapy, the sleep disorder may disappear. Otherwise, chloral hydrate in doses of 250 mg to 1 gm is an effective hypnotic; it's preferred over barbiturates, which can cause confusion and paradoxical agitation. Flurazepam HCl (Dalmane) is a useful hypnotic that produces little suppression of REM sleep.

Tolerance to hypnotics can develop, and, like all CNS depressants, hypnotics induce hepatic microsomal enzymes into speeding the metabolism of simultaneously administered drugs. Except for flurazepam, hypnotics depress REM sleep, which can cause hallucinations and insomnia when the drug is discontinued.

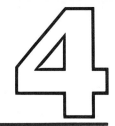

Tailoring Cardiovascular Therapy to the Patient

By Fred S. Gordon, R.Ph., M.S.

Elderly patients are especially susceptible to heart failure, high blood pressure, and blood clot formation in peripheral and cerebral vessels. Potent drugs are available for treating these disorders, but alterations brought on by age in renal function, metabolic rates, absorption, and distribution can easily lead to toxic effects and adverse reactions.

Four major types of cardiovascular drugs—digitalis glycosides, diuretics, coronary vasodilators, and antihypertensive agents—are represented in the accompanying tables. The tables include modifications in drug dosages to prevent toxic effects and adverse reactions in aging patients, routes and times of administration, problems to be alert for, and the treatment implications of each drug.

59

DIGITALIS GLYCOSIDES   Monitor for toxicity and hypokalemia.

Have defibrillation and cardiac pacing equipment on hand during digitalization.

Give drugs near meals to minimize gastric distress.

Count the pulse for a full minute before administering the drug.

Physician must be called if the pulse is 60 or below, or the rate, rhythm, or quality changes.

Drug	Indications	Adult and geriatric dosages	Treatment implications
Digitalis	Congestive heart failure, atrial fibrillation, atrial flutter, paroxysmal atrial tachycardia	**Adult**—Digitalizing: 50-150 mg P.O. t.i.d.-q.i.d. for 3-4 days to maximum of 1 gm. Maintenance: 100 mg q.d. Onset of action 1-2 hours, duration 1-3 days. **Geriatric**—Reduced for renal impairment, hypokalemia, metabolic anomaly	Serves as a prototype for the glycosides. Onset of action is slow and duration prolonged. Maximal effects 6-8 hours after administration. Action regresses in 2-3 days and disappears in 2-3 weeks.
Digitoxin	Congestive heart failure, atrial fibrillation, atrial flutter, paroxysmal atrial tachycardia	**Adult**—Digitalizing: 1.0-1.5 mg P.O., I.M., or I.V. one-third to one-half in the initial dose and one-eighth to one-third q3-6h or 200 mcg b.i.d. for 4 days. Maintenance: 50-300 mcg q.d. Onset of action 25 minutes-2 hours, maximum effect 4-12 hours, duration 2-3 weeks. **Geriatric**—Reduced for renal impairment, hypokalemia, metabolic anomaly	Don't confuse with digoxin. Most potent of digitalis glycosides. Unsuitable for emergencies. S.C. injection unsuitable and may be irritating. Inject deeply into gluteal muscle. Drug is eliminated slowly.

Drug	Indications	Adult and geriatric dosages	Treatment implications
Digoxin	Congestive heart failure, atrial fibrillation, atrial flutter, paroxysmal atrial tachycardia	**Adult**—Digitalizing: 2-3 mg I.M. or P.O., one-fourth to one-half in the initial dose and the remainder divided q6h for 24 hours; I.V. 0.5-1.0 mg q2-4h as required. Maintenance: 0.25-0.75 mg q.d. Onset of action 5-30 minutes, maximum effect 2-5 hours, duration 2-6 days. **Geriatric**—Digitalizing: 0.5-1.5 mg in 24 hours. Maintenance: 0.125-0.25 mg q.d.	Don't confuse with digitoxin. Shorter duration than digitoxin and digitalis. In severe congestive heart failure, absorption of I.M. injection may be delayed. Effect may be prolonged. Inject deeply into muscle and follow with vigorous massage. Rotate injection sites.
Ouabain	Rapid digitalization in emergency treatment of atrial flutter, atrial fibrillation, and paroxysmal tachycardia	**Adult**—Digitalizing: 1 mg I.V. with initial dose of 0.25 mg and the remainder in doses of 0.1-0.25 mg q30-60 minutes. Onset of action 3-10 minutes, maximum effect 30-60 minutes, duration 1-3 days. **Geriatric**—Reduced for renal impairment	Emergency use only. Don't give the drug to patients who have received digitalis during previous 3 weeks.
Lanatoside C (Cedilanid)	Congestive heart failure, atrial fibrillation, atrial flutter, paroxysmal atrial tachycardia	**Adult**—Digitalizing: 8-10 mg P.O. 3.5 mg on day 1, 2.5 mg on day 2, 2.0 mg daily on succeeding days as required. Maintenance: 0.5-1.5 mg q.d. Duration 16 hours-3 days. **Geriatric**—Reduced for renal impairment	Don't give the drug to patients who have received digitalis during previous 2 weeks. Protect container from light. Rarely given to geriatric patients because of poor absorption from the G.I. tract.

DIURETICS (Thiazide)

Drug	Indications	Adult and geriatric dosages	Treatment implications
Chlorothiazide	Edema and hypertension	**Adult**—0.5-1.0 gm P.O. q.d.-b.i.d. for edema, 250 mg b.i.d.-500 mg t.i.d. for hypertension. **Geriatric**—Titrated to renal function and condition	Administer before noon to prevent nocturia and with food to prevent G.I. irritation. Be aware of possible increase in incontinence in geriatric patients. Explain the effects to the patient. The intake-output ratio must be accounted for, and the drug discontinued if oliguria develops. Possibility of orthostatic hypotension is increased. Pre-existing diabetes mellitus may be aggravated. Monitor serum levels of glucose, potassium, chloride, sodium, BUN, NPN, uric acid, and bicarbonate. Discontinue the drug 1 week before elective surgery.
Hydrochlorothiazide	Edema and hypertension	**Adult**—25-100 mg P.O. q.d.-b.i.d. for edema, 25-50 mg q.d.-b.i.d. for hypertension. **Geriatric**—Titrated to renal function	
Polythiazide (Renese)	Edema and hypertension	**Adult and geriatric**—1-4 mg P.O. q.d. for edema and hypertension. Duration up to 36 hours	

DIURETICS (Other types)

Drug	Indications	Adult and geriatric dosages	Treatment implications
Acetazolamide (Diamox)	Edema, epilepsy, glaucoma, emphysema	**Adult and geriatric**—250-375 mg P.O., I.V., or I.M. every morning or every other morning for edema	Tolerance after prolonged use may necessitate dosage increase. I.M. route painful. Paresthesia and drowsiness common. See thiazide precautions.

Drug	Indications	Adult and geriatric dosages	Treatment implications
Chlorthalidone	Edema and hypertension	**Adult**—50-100 mg P.O. q.d. initially, then 100 mg 3 times a week. **Geriatric**—Titrated to renal function and need	Give in the morning with food. Particularly good for potentiating action and reducing dosage of other hypotensive agents.
Ethacrynic acid (Edecrin)	Edema and hypertension	**Adult**—50 mg P.O. after breakfast of day 1, 50 mg after breakfast and lunch of day 2, 100 mg after breakfast and 50-100 mg after lunch and evening meal of day 3. 400 mg maximum daily dose thereafter. **Geriatric**—Titrated to renal function and need	Always give after meals. Observe patient for excessive diuresis (more than 2-pound daily weight loss). Electrolyte imbalance more likely at higher rates of diuresis. Potassium supplement may be necessary. Watch for bloody stools and hematuria. Discontinue drug if diarrhea is excessive.
Furosemide (Lasix)	Edema and hypertension	**Adult and geriatric**—40-80 mg P.O. q.d. increased by 40 mg q6-8h in resistant cases for edema, 40 mg P.O. (I.M. or I.V. if necessary) b.i.d. for hypertension	Potent drug. Monitor blood pressure closely. Be alert for signs of hypokalemia, dehydration, and circulatory collapse, vascular thrombosis, and embolism, particularly in the elderly. Assure patient that pain after I.M. injection is transient. Give aspirin with caution. Diuresis may be accompanied by weakness, fatigue, lightheadedness, dizziness, perspiration, muscle cramps, bladder spasm, and feeling of urgency.

Drug	Indications	Adult and geriatric dosages	Treatment implications
Mannitol	Edema	**Adult**—Test dose 200 mg/kg I.V. in 2-5 minutes. 24-hour dosage 50-100 gm. **Geriatric**—Titrated to individual need	Be alert for chest pain. Relieve thirst and provide fluids only in controlled conditions. Adequate response is 40 ml urine/hour (2-3 hours).
Quinethazone (Hydromox)	Edema and hypertension	**Adult and geriatric**—50-100 mg P.O. q.d. For maintenance, adjust to response	Long-acting sulfonamide having the same activity and side effects as the thiazides. May precipitate gout.
Spironolactone (Aldactone)	Edema	**Adult**—100 mg P.O. q.d. in divided doses for at least 5 days, with dosage then adjusted according to response. **Geriatric**—Titrated to renal function and need	See thiazide precautions. Spares potassium so supplements aren't necessary. Large doses may cause ataxia and drowsiness. Tolerance to drug, characterized by edema and reduction in urine output, may develop. Watch for stupor and coma in patients with history of liver disease. Monitor blood pressure daily. Adjust dosage or discontinue the drug if oliguria develops.
Theobromine calcium salicylate	Edema	**Adult**—0.5-1.0 gm P.O. t.i.d. after meals. **Geriatric**—Titrated to need, but rarely ordered	See thiazide precautions. Observe for cumulative effect in patients receiving drug more frequently than q8h. Possible side effects include headache, nervousness, dizziness, insomnia, and palpitations.

Drug	Indications	Adult and geriatric dosages	Treatment implications
Triamterene (Dyazide, Dyrenium)	Edema and hypertension	**Adult and geriatric**—100 mg P.O. q.d.-b.i.d. initially, then 100 mg every other day for edema. 100 mg b.i.d. after meals usually with a thiazide for hypertension	See thiazide precautions. Spares potassium, so supplements usually not necessary. Potassium may be retained, so avoid potassium-rich foods. Possible side effects include blood dyscrasias (sore throat, fever, rash) and uremia (lethargy, headache, drowsiness, vomiting, restlessness, mental wandering, and foul breath). Give after meals to minimize stomach upset.
Urea	Edema	**Adult**—1 gm/kg I.V. over 2-2.5 hours to a maximum of 120 gm in 24 hours. **Geriatrics**—Titrated to individual need	See thiazide precautions. May increase effects of anticoagulants. Don't administer into lower extremities of geriatric patients because the drug has a fibrinolytic effect. Observe congestive heart failure patients carefully. Monitor vital signs, as increase in plasma volume by drug may precipitate pulmonary edema.

CORONARY VASODILATORS

Instruct patients carrying sublingual tablets to observe the expiration date on bottle and to obtain a fresh bottle when needed.

Instruct patient to sit or lie down to take sublingual tablet to prevent postural hypotension.

The hospitalized patient should be allowed to keep this medication at his bedside, but be aware of how much drug he needs to relieve his angina, how frequently the patient takes the drug, whether relief is partial or complete, the length of time before relief is attained, and whether side effects occur. Chart all observations.

Observe patients for signs of tolerance. Nitrites may be discontinued until tolerance subsides.

Patients taking nitrites should be aware of dangerous interactions with alcohol. Nitrite syncope, a severe shocklike state, may occur.

Observe for nausea, headache, vomiting, drowsiness, and visual disturbances during long-term prophylaxis.

Observe for sensitivity to hypotensive effect such as nausea, pallor, restlessness, and collapse.

Observe for potentiating effects of other hypotensive drugs used as additional therapy.

Drug	Indications	Adult and geriatric dosages	Treatment implications
Amyl nitrite	Angina	**Adult and geriatric**—0.18-0.3 ml inhaled from crushed ampule	The fabric-covered ampule is to be enclosed in a handkerchief or cloth and crushed by hand. Warn the patient that the drug has a strong and pungent odor, but that he is to take several deep breaths of it nevertheless. Amyl nitrite is flammable.

Drug	Indications	Adult and geriatric dosages	Treatment implications
Erythrityl tetranitrate (Cardilate)	Coronary insufficiency	**Adult and geriatric**—5-15 mg sublingual, 10-30 mg P.O. t.i.d.	A tingling sensation may occur at the site of lingual administration. Watch for vascular headaches and G.I. disturbances. Use analgesic to relieve headaches. Not suitable for acute attacks.
Isosorbide dinitrate	Coronary insufficiency	**Adult and geriatric**—5-30 mg P.O. q.i.d. Prophylaxis 5-10 mg sublingual as tolerated	To be taken with meals to reduce or eliminate headaches. Not preferred for acute attacks.
Mannitol hexanitrate	Coronary insufficiency	**Adult and geriatric**—32-64 gm P.O. q4-6h	Observe for respiratory distress. Check blood pressure at least twice a day for hypotension. Be alert for complaints of headache. Observe for shock symptoms indicating cardiovascular collapse.
Nitroglycerin	Angina	**Adult and geriatric**—300-600 mcg sublingual q2-3h as required, 400 mcg q5minutes for acute attack until pain is relieved	Drug of choice. Tablets should be stored in the original tightly closed glass container. Tablets that don't cause a local burning sensation have probably deteriorated.
Pentaerythritol tetranitrate	Coronary insufficiency	**Adult and geriatric**—10-30 mg P.O. before meals and at bedtime	Not used sublingually. For prophylaxis.

ANTIHYPERTENSIVE AGENTS

Drug	Indications	Adult and geriatric dosages	Treatment implications
Diazoxide (Hyperstat-I.V.)	Hypertensive crisis	**Adult and geriatric**—300 mg or 5 mg/kg I.V. rapidly injected	Protect drug from light, heat, and freezing. Have the patient recumbent during and for 30 minutes after injection. Have patient recumbent for 8-10 hours if furosemide is used as part of therapy. Closely monitor blood pressure after injection, until stable, and then every hour. Check final blood pressure when the patient is standing. Check for glycosuria.
Hydralazine HCl	Early malignant hypertension	**Adult**—10-25 mg P.O. q.d. increased if necessary to 200 mg divided into 4 doses; 10-20 mg I.M. or I.V. q.d. increased to 40 mg if necessary. **Geriatric**—Titrated to individual need and renal function	Administer P.O. to ambulatory patients at bedtime for those with moderate to severe hypertension. Blood pressure may fall within 5-10 minutes after parenteral injection. Observe for influenza-type reaction early during therapy, or a rheumatoid syndrome which may necessitate discontinuing drug. Watch for postural hypotension. Warn the patient to sit or lie down if he feels weak or dizzy. Take blood pressure several times a day and 5 minutes after parenteral injection.

Drug	Indications	Adult and geriatric dosages	Treatment implications
Guanethidine sulfate (Ismelin)	Hypertension, thiazide-induced edema	**Adult outpatient**—10 mg P.O. q.d. initially, then increased by 10 mg each week to maintenance dose of 25-50 mg q.d.; **Hospital patients**—25-50 mg q.d. as needed. **Geriatric**—Titrated to individual need	Watch for postural hypotension. Warn the patient to sit or lie down if he feels weak or dizzy. Report bradycardia and diarrhea to the physician. Monitor blood pressure, pulse, and intake and output. Patients on therapy for stress may incur cardiovascular collapse. Monitor accordingly.
Methyldopa	Hypertension	**Adult**—250 mg P.O. b.i.d. for 2 days and then adjusted. Maximum dose 3 gm q.d. **Geriatric**—Titrated to individual need	Watch for postural hypotension. Observe for signs of tolerance. Weigh patient daily, observing for signs of edema. Monitor intake and output, and observe for reduced urine output. Sedation may occur with initial therapy, but will usually disappear when maintenance dose is established. In rare cases, urine may darken or turn blue. The reaction is not harmful.

Drug	Indications	Adult and geriatric dosages	Treatment implications
Reserpine	Mild to moderate hypertension	**Adult**—0.25-0.5 mg P.O. q.d. initially, then 0.1-0.25 mg. 1-5 mg parenterally q6-12 h. **Geriatric**—0.25-0.5 mg P.O. q.d. as maintenance dose	Even with low doses, fluid retention and/or parkinsonism may result. Because of the high incidence of drug-induced depression, reserpine should be used in the geriatric patients only for mild cases of hypertension requiring low doses. Watch for personality changes, depression, and complaints of nightmares. Postural hypotension and respiratory depression may occur. Take blood pressure and pulse before each administration. Supervise ambulation. Administer after meals to reduce gastric distress.

OTC Drugs and the Elderly

By Peter P. Lamy, Ph.D.

Nonprescription drugs can contribute importantly to patient well-being. However, certain agents, such as aspirin, vitamins, and antacids, can cause serious adverse reactions as well as additive effects and interactions with prescription drugs.[1,2] Since the reactions of these drugs seem particularly enhanced in the elderly, it's important to question these patients closely regarding their use of OTCs and to carefully document and monitor this usage.

Self-treatment

Selection of a particular OTC drug based on self-diagnosis may be erroneous, and self-treatment may lead to unfortunate clinical consequences. For example, the persistent use of cough remedies can delay diagnosis of a serious respiratory illness. And the failure to follow label instructions can lead to overdosage with an OTC drug that contains ingredients usually available in equivalent amounts only on prescription.

Unfortunately, it's friends and relatives, rather than health professionals, who probably have primary influence over a patient's self-medication habits, making the appropriate use of these drugs questionable.[3] So far, physicians have had little influence on OTC drug usage,[4] a situation that should be corrected.

Incidence of OTC drug use

The incidence of acute conditions—those for which nonprescription drugs are most often used—declines sharply with age. The incidence of other conditions—arthritis, gastrointestinal problems, sinusitis—increases with age, and OTC drug usage is heavy among patients with these disorders. According to one study, persons between 17 and 44 years of age had 282 acute conditions (including multiple incidents) per 100 persons per year; for those 65 years and older, the rate was only 102 acute conditions.[5] It's interesting that the age-specific rates for women exceed those for men throughout the life-span and that, although we're not sure why, women, particularly whites, are most prone to adverse drug reactions.

Individually, the elderly have a high number of visits to office-based general and family practitioners, as compared to younger patients[6]; back problems, throat soreness, abdominal pain, cough, cold, and headache rank high among their primary complaints. As these problems can be managed with OTC drugs, there are probably many more elderly patients with similar complaints who do not visit a physician.

These minor complaints, if not cared for and thus allowed to linger, tend to develop into major health problems in the elderly. And, although the elderly experience fewer acute conditions than do younger persons, the effects of these minor problems are more serious and result in longer disability.[5] Additionally, the elderly may use OTC drugs to self-treat chronic conditions—arthritic pain is one of the major reasons for OTC analgesic use among these patients.[7]

The most often used OTCs are vitamins, analgesics, cold remedies, and laxatives. In one study, almost 50 per cent of elderly

Major OTC/Rx drug interactions

OTC drug	Rx drug	Effects
Acetaminophen (8 tablets/day)	Anticoagulants, coumarin	Slightly increased hypoprothrombinemic response
	Antihypertensives	Possibility of severe hypertensive reaction or hypertensive episode
Antacids		
Aluminum, magnesium	Indomethacin (Indocin)	Decreased GI absorption and effect of indomethacin
Aluminum	Isoniazid	Decreased GI absorption and effect of isoniazid
Aluminum, calcium, magnesium	Tetracyclines, oral	Impaired absorption and decreased effect of tetracycline
Iron	Tetracyclines	Impaired GI absorption, decreased serum levels, and decreased effect of tetracycline
Kaolin-pectin	Digitalis	Reduced serum levels and effect of digitalis
	Lincomycin (Lincocin)	Serum concentrations of lincomycin reduced by 90%; decreased effect of lincomycin
Laxatives, phenolphthalein	Anticoagulants	Increased hypoprothrombinemia

OTC drug	Rx drug	Effects
Salicylates < 2 gm/day	Anticoagulants	Possibility of impaired primary hemostasis; GI bleeding
Salicylates > 2 gm/day	Anticoagulants	Enhanced hypoprothrombinemic effect
	Oral hypoglycemics	Increased hypoglycemia; enhanced hypoglycemic response to sulfonylureas
	Methotrexate	Decreased clearance of methotrexate; decreased plasma protein binding; increased methotrexate toxicity
	Probenecid (Benemid)	Decreased uricosuric effect
Sympathomimetics (in most cold and cough preparations)	Antihypertensives	Decreased antihypertensive effect
	Digitalis	Increased possibility of cardiac arrhythmias
Vitamin A	Anticoagulants	Inhibition of anticoagulant effect
Vitamin C (ascorbic acid)	Anticoagulants	Altered anticoagulant effect
Vitamin E	Anticoagulants	Enhanced hypoprothrombinemic response; interference with effect of vitamin K in producing clotting factors

persons self-administered vitamins.[8] Another group found that more than two-thirds of elderly ambulatory patients used OTC drugs.[9] More than half of these drugs were oral analgesics; cough and cold preparations accounted for about 13 per cent. However, only 8 per cent of the patients surveyed felt they needed an OTC drug to perform regular daily activities, and only 12 per cent consulted a physician about their OTC drug use. Moreover, the elderly may use almost twice as many OTC preparations as prescription products— 7.25 vs. 3.8 in one study—with oral analgesics and gastrointestinal agents used most often.[10] However, another group found that OTC drug use among noninstitutionalized elderly closely paralleled that of prescription drugs.[11]

Nonprescription drug use is also high among institutionalized elderly patients. Laxatives, oral analgesics, antacids, and vitamins are among those most frequently administered in long-term care facilities.[4] Furthermore, nonprescription drugs may possibly be used more frequently than prescription drugs in rural areas.[12] Socioeconomic factors also influence drug use patterns. Vitamin supplements are more likely to be used by higher-income persons, while digestive remedies appear to be more popular among lower-income groups.

One must be aware of the clinical consequences that can result from unnecessary or chronic OTC drug usage. Of more than 4,000 drug abuse studies performed on the elderly between 1926 and 1975, 10 per cent dealt with the adverse effects related to inappropriate OTC usage.[5] Adverse effects include the development of renal tumors, pyelonephritis, GI bleeding, and abnormal thyroid function.[13]

Vitamins

Inadequate intake of vitamins A, B_1, thiamine, B_2, B_6, B_{12}, C (ascorbic acid), D, and E, as well as of niacin and folic acid, has been demonstrated among the elderly.[14] This is not surprising: A diet of fewer than 2,000 calories per day isn't likely to supply their vitamin needs, and calorie intake declines with increasing age.

Although reduced calorie intake is desirable as energy expenditure also declines, the decrease may be excessive because of poor dentition, a lack of saliva, and a decrease in the number and efficiency of taste buds. In addition, many older persons can't afford a well-balanced diet. Lack of interest in cooking and social isolation also contribute to vitamin deficiencies.

Such deficiencies, often subclinical, may be clinically significant in patients with a newly diagnosed acute disease. It's been suggested that mortality increases among elderly persons deficient in vitamins, particularly vitamin A, niacin, and ascorbic acid.[15]

On the other hand, excessive vitamin intake can lead to unanticipated clinical consequences. Large doses of vitamins A and D can be toxic. It's also possible that excess thiamine adversely affects the cardiovascular and nervous systems. Too much niacin can be responsible for abnormal liver function and high levels of uric acid and glucose, while excessive folic acid may lead to toxicities involving the central nervous and renal systems. Megadoses of vitamin C may cause precipitation of cystine and oxalate stones and may shorten prothrombin time when heparin or warfarin is used. Large doses of vitamin E—often taken in the belief that it will slow the aging process—may enhance the action of warfarin.

Since vitamins can also interfere with many laboratory test results, patients should stop taking supplements before certain tests, such as alkaline phosphatase, bilirubin, calcium, cholesterol, and occult blood tests, are performed. Vitamin C, for example, can cause a false-negative result on the occult blood test.

There has been much dispute as to whether vitamin supplementation for the elderly is warranted when there's no clear-cut evidence of deficiency. Yet, when viewed in terms of risk vs. benefit, it seems that the potential benefit considerably outweights any possible complication if supplementation is closely supervised.

Select for your patients a vitamin formula that supplies the basic needs of water- and fat-soluble vitamins; added minerals and trace metals appear necessary only in cases of frank deficiency.

I have to wonder about the often-cited excessive use of iron among the elderly, as hemoglobin and serum levels—at least among the noninstitutionalized—do not seem to vary significantly from those of younger populations.[16] Explain that too much of a good thing can be harmful, and caution patients against taking more than the recommended dosage.

Cough and cold remedies

The common cold is a self-limiting respiratory condition. OTC cough and cold preparations help provide some relief—usually temporary—from its symptoms. However, physicians should warn elderly pa-

Salicylate influence on some lab test values

Laboratory test	Results
Blood	
Benedict's test	Elevated levels→false-positive
Carbon dioxide	Elevated levels→false-positive Decreased levels→false-negative
Cholesterol	Decreased levels→false-negative
Fasting glucose	Decreased levels→false-negative
Glucose	Elevated levels→false-positive
Platelets	Decreased levels→false-negative
Potassium	Decreased levels→false-negative
Protein-bound iodine (PBI)	Decreased levels→false-negative
Prothrombin time	Elevated levels→false-positive
Triiodothyronine (T_3) uptake	Elevated levels→false-positive (when salicylates given in high doses)
Uric acid	Elevated levels→false-positive (when not done by enzymatic method)

Laboratory test	Results
CSF	
Proteins in spinal fluid (Folin-Ciocalteu method)	Elevated levels→false-positive
Urine	
Diacetic acid	Elevated levels→false-positive
Glucose	Possibly false-positive or false-negative (with moderate to high doses)
Phenylketone	Possibly false-positive or false-negative
Proteins	Elevated levels→false-positive
Uric acid	Elevated levels→false-positive

tients that these preparations are designed to treat coughs associated with self-limiting conditions and *not* chronic problems. Explain that relieving the cough in certain conditions, such as asthma or emphysema, can result in retention of respiratory secretions and can be harmful. Additionally, encourage patients to report any cold, so you can determine whether it's merely a cold or the symptom of something more serious.

Nearly all cold preparations contain a sympathomimetic amine, such as phenylephrine or phenylpropanolamine, that acts as a bronchodilator or decongestant. Some of these products may cause nervousness, dizziness, or insomnia. Tell your elderly patients that these products may be contraindicated if they have high blood pressure, are taking antidepressant medication, are diabetic, or have a thyroid condition. Some preparations also contain antihistamines; advise elderly patients with asthma, glaucoma, or an enlarged prostate gland against usage.

Anticholinergics are often included in cold preparations to inhibit excessive tearing and "runny nose." Elderly patients may be particularly susceptible to the side effects of these agents if they have an underlying disease state, such as asthma, prostate enlargement, or angle-closure glaucoma; these patients should avoid using anticholinergic-containing products.

Also at increased risk of side effects from these preparations are patients already receiving one or more drugs with anticholinergic action, such as phenothiazines, antiparkinsonism drugs, or tricyclic antidepressants. Explain that they should discontinue any anticholinergic OTCs when confusion, constipation, rapid pulse, or blurred vision occur. Alert family members to the possibility of these side effects; a confused patient may not notice these reactions.

Laxatives

About 50 per cent of all elderly persons probably use laxatives, with those over the age of 70 taking them twice as often as those between 40 and 50 years of age.[17]

This high usage is probably not reasonable, although a multitude of mechanical, physiologic, and psychologic conditions in the elderly can predispose them to constipation.

Poor dentition is often cited as a factor in constipation, as it leads to poor nutritional intake—both qualitative and quantitative.

Inadequate fluid intake, particularly by incontinent patients, and lack of exercise, especially in bed-bound patients, contribute to the problem. Diverticular disease, neurologic disease, cancer, fissures, or hemorrhoids may be factors, as well as hypokalemia, hypothyroidism, hypercalcemia, depression, or stress.

Not infrequently, constipation is caused by drugs, such as ganglionic blockers, tricyclic antidepressants, antihistamines, antiparkinsonism drugs, and phenothiazines. Other agents that can cause constipation include antacids containing aluminum or calcium carbonate, iron salts, and opiates.

Thus, laxative selection should be based on a careful evaluation of the individual patient and the causes of his constipation, giving due consideration to differences in laxative efficacy and to the incidence of side effects. We must also remember that habitual laxative usage may contribute to constipation. Irritant laxatives can provoke a "cathartic colon" or the irritable bowel syndrome. Watery diarrhea, weight loss, and weakness may be signs of long-term intake of large doses. On the other hand, laxative use may be indicated when it's impossible to retrain a chronically abused, malfunctioning, dyskinetic colon.

Bulk laxatives are indicated when a constipating, low-residue diet can't be corrected—because of noncompliance, for example—but are contraindicated in the presence of strictures of the colon. These laxatives should be administered with large volumes (at least 8 ounces) of water to avoid intestinal obstruction. Effervescent forms, which contain large amounts of sodium, may be contraindicated in persons on low-salt diets; stool softeners are probably indicated only for patients with normal intestinal tone who have dry, hard stools.

Among the saline laxatives, milk of magnesia is probably the safest and most widely used. (To work effectively, it should be taken with at least 8 ounces of water.) The major hazard of saline laxatives is the possibility of electrolyte disturbance. Similarly, excessive use of stimulant laxatives can lead to electrolyte disturbances, particularly hypokalemia. For this reason, castor oil is not indicated in elderly patients.

Antacids

Antacids are widely used by the general population. Potency, palatability, and sodium content are among the factors to consider when selecting a particular product for the elderly. Also remember that elderly patients may not be able to handle a comparatively heavy bottle, and that liquid products are suspensions and must be well shaken. If elderly patients switch to tablets, treatment failure may result, as this dosage may not provide the same effectiveness as suspensions. Activity largely depends on surface area. Even if patients were to chew tablets vigorously, they can't achieve the same surface area as they can with liquids.

Palatability may be especially important for elderly patients and can determine whether they comply with a particular regimen. Antacids containing calcium carbonate can produce acid rebound and have constipating properties. These products should therefore be used with caution in elderly patients complaining of constipation.

Aluminum hydroxide, also constipating, is most frequently marketed in products that contain magnesium salts to offset this property. Intestinal obstruction in elderly patients—particularly those with decreased bowel motility, as in bedridden patients or those on restricted fluid intake—is possible with aluminum-containing antacids, but usually not with preparations containing both aluminum and magnesium.

Salicylate/Rx drug interactions

Rx drug	Effect with salicylate
Aminosalicylic acid	Increased possibility of salicylate toxicity
Anticoagulants	Enhanced anticoagulant effect, especially with salicylate doses > 1 gm/day
Corticosteroids	Increased possibility of GI ulceration
Methotrexate	Possible methotrexate displacement from albumin binding sites; increased toxicity
Phenobarbital	Decreased effect of salicylates due to enzyme induction
Phenylbutazone	Increased possibility of GI ulceration; inhibition of uricosuria; possible competition for plasma protein binding
Phenytoin	Enhanced anticonvulsant activity with large doses of salicylate due to displacement from plasma protein binding sites
Probenecid (Benemid)	Altered uricosuric activity of probenecid
Sulfonylureas	Enhanced hypoglycemic response

Sodium retention following antacid use may be of clinical consequence if the patient takes sodium-containing antacids in large doses or has decreased renal function. Effervescent preparations and those with sodium bicarbonate usually contain a large amount of sodium. Those OTC antacids containing more than 0.2 mEq (5 mg) of sodium per dose must now carry an appropriate cautionary note on the label.

Several important interactions involving antacids can occur. Antacids increase absorption of acidic drugs and decrease absorption of basic drugs. By delaying gastric emptying, antacids delay the absorption of drugs, such as imipramine HCl, meperidine HCl (Demerol), and quinine, that are primarily absorbed from the intestine.

Also, antacids can influence the elimination processes of some drugs by affecting urinary pH. When an elderly patient complains of constipation, nausea, upset stomach, or other gastrointestinal problems, remember that excessive antacid intake may be responsible.

Analgesics

Because the elderly frequently use OTC analgesics, it's important to remember the following:

• Pain is a warning signal; it's necessary to discover the cause of pain, as well as to alleviate it.

• Persistent use of analgesics can alleviate early warning symptoms and delay diagnosis of a serious problem.

• Various analgesics are contraindicated in patients taking certain prescription drugs.

Aspirin is unquestionably the most frequently used of all OTC drugs. It's relatively inexpensive, easily accessible, and has analgesic, anti-inflammatory, and antipyretic actions—there's no better OTC analgesic. However, large doses of aspirin can produce gastrointestinal irritation, and the frequency and amount of gastrointestinal bleeding can be clinically significant in the elderly. High doses also produce a decrease in sodium and chloride excretion.

Indiscriminate usage can lead to toxicity, which appears at lower dose levels in the elderly. The drug's half-life increases with the dose, as does toxicity. When the dose is lowered, toxic effects usually decline and disappear. Signs and symptoms of salicylate toxicity include confusion, irritability, tinnitus, hearing and vision disturbances, sweating, nausea, vomiting, and diarrhea. Since many of these symptoms are inappropriately ascribed to old age, toxicity may be overlooked by both the patient and the provider—physician or pharmacist.

Aspirin's antipyretic action can cause subnormal temperatures in the elderly; chronic rheumatism patients on long-term aspirin therapy frequently complain of shivering and feeling cold. Combined use of aspirin and other drugs that upset the thermoregulatory mechanism could lead to hypothermia.

As shown in the accompanying tables, salicylates influence many laboratory test values and interact with a number of prescription drugs. Therefore, while aspirin is an almost indispensable drug for the elderly, usage should be closely monitored by physicians and pharmacists.

Greater awareness of aspirin's potential adverse effects has led to a substantial increase in the use of acetaminophen. With similar analgesic and antipyretic properties, acetaminophen is a suitable substitute for aspirin when required for these purposes. At the recommended dose—650 mg q4 to 6h—it doesn't produce gastric irritation, erosion, or occult blood loss. Acetaminophen is generally preferred for patients receiving oral anticoagulants and for those with hyperuricemia, gouty arthritis, asthma, or peptic ulcer.

Aspirin, on the other hand, is far superior in the management of rheumatoid arthritis; it has an anti-inflammatory action that acetaminophen lacks. Acetaminophen is not effective in treating severe pain of any kind. Overdoses can lead to serious hepatotoxicity. Acetaminophen is also much costlier than aspirin.

References

1. Lamy PP, Kitler ME: Untoward effects of drugs: I (including nonprescription drugs). *Dis Nerv Syst* 32:17, 1971
2. Lamy PP, Kitler ME: Untoward effects of drugs: II (including nonprescription drugs). *Dis Nerv Syst* 32:105, 1971
3. Purnell J: Analgesic consumption in a country town. *Med J Aust* 8:389, 1967
4. Lamy PP (ed): *Prescribing for the Elderly*, ch 15. Littleton, Mass: PSG Publishing, 1979
5. Black ER: Acute conditions: Incidence and associated disability, US, July 1976-June 1977. DHEW Publ No (PHS) 78-1553. Hyattsville, Md: National Center for Health Statistics, 1978
6. Cypress BK: National ambulatory medical care survey of visits to general and family practitioners, January-December 1975. *Advancedata* 15:1, 1977
7. Matte DA, McLean WM: Self-medication abuse or misuse? *Drug Intelligence & Clinical Pharmacy* 12:603, 1978
8. Rose CS, Gyorgy P, Butler M, et al: Age differences in vitamin B-6 status of 617 men. *Am J Clin Nutr* 29:847, 1976

9. Guttman D: A survey of drug-taking behavior of older Americans. In *Medication Management and Education of the Elderly* (Beber CR and Lamy PP, eds) p 18. Princeton, NJ: Excerpta Medica, 1978

10. Boykin SP, de Paul Burkhart VP, Lamy PP: Drug use in a day treatment center. *Am J Hosp Pharm* 35:155, 1978

11. Vener AM, Krupka LR, Climo JJ: Drug usage and health characteristics in noninstitutional retired persons. *J Am Geriatr Soc* 27:83, 1979

12. Salber FJ, Greene SB, Gagnon JP, et al: Black/white drug use pattern in rural North Carolina. *Contemporary Pharmacy Practice* 2:4, 1979

13. Report prepared by Science Information Services, Franklin Institute Research Laboratories, Philadelphia, Pa, under contract No. ADM-NIDA 74-117. Rockville, Md: National Institute on Drug Abuse, Public Health Service, 1975

14. Preliminary Findings of the First Health and Nutrition Examination Survey, US, 1971-1972: Dietary intake and biochemical findings. DHEW Publ No (HRA) 74-1219-1. Hyattsville, Md: National Center for Health Statistics, 1974

15. Brin M, Bauernfeind JC: Vitamin needs of the elderly. *Postgrad Med* 63:155, 1978

16. Johnson CL, Abraham S: Hemoglobin and selected iron related findings of persons 1-74 years of age: US, 1971-74. *Advancedata* 46:1, 1979

17. Berman PM, Kirsner JB: Gastrointestinal problems. In *Cowdrey's The Care of the Geriatric Patient* (Steinberg FU, ed), 5th ed, p 103. St. Louis: CV Mosby, 1976

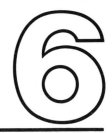

Medication Mistakes and Noncompliance

Of equal importance to understanding how drugs act in elderly patients are knowing what are the ways the elderly manipulate—willfully or by accident—their drug diets and knowing how to correct their mistakes.

All people deviate from a prescribed regimen, if only to miss a dose now and then. But the elderly are far more likely to misuse or fail to use medications.

Many older people live alone and are depressed, disinclined to take measures that will keep them alive longer, and resigned to "suffering" the effects of aging. Some may have developed inadequate health habits, and some may prefer self-medication with nonprescription drugs that have become their favorite remedies for a **93** host of disorders. They may be unaware that, in many cases, modern drugs can control chronic disorders and significantly improve the quality of their lives. Finally, many don't want to face dependence on drugs or the drain on their retirement dollars that medical treatment entails.

Drug abuse

Together with swapping stories about their disorders, some elderly readily offer their friends leftover medications that "worked just fine" for them when they had symptoms similar to what their friends describe. And they just as readily accept others' medications, without regard for what other disorders they may have or what other drugs they are taking, in combination with which these borrowed drugs can cause great harm.

Some older patients feel free to increase the dosage if they haven't felt a drug's effect after a couple of days, unaware that that may be the way the drug acts. The same simple way of viewing how drugs work is operative in the person who makes up for a missed dose by doubling the next one.

Some patients with acute illnesses stop their medication on their own, cutting short the full course of treatment, because they feel better and think the drug has done its work. A patient with a chronic disorder may reduce the dosage to make the prescribed amount of medicine last longer. A patient who does this fails to attain a therapeutic level of the drug, and the "longer-lasting" medicine, used after its expiration date, may have lost its potency.

Medication mistakes that are potentially more dangerous than these are mistakes that result in adverse reactions or drug interactions. Some of these are caused by patients, some are iatrogenic, and some are out of anyone's control until they occur, results of particular somatic conditions that affect absorption and excretion of drugs. The last of these are described in other chapters of this book.

Eighty per cent of the over-60 have a chronic disorder, and a significant number of them—35 per cent—have three or more. The patient with multiple disorders, of course, is subject to polypharmacy, even if he is in the care of only one physician. The problem is compounded if the patient sees more than one physician, gets his drugs at more than one pharmacy, and tells no one what the others are prescribing or dispensing. Taking more than one drug may dimin-

Foods that foil drugs

Eleanor Bauwens, R.N., Ph.D., and Cindy Clemmons, R.N., B.S.N.

If your patient takes:	And eats or drinks:	The combination may:	So intervene to:
Acetaminophen	Carbohydrates	Retard the absorption rate of the drug, though not the total amount absorbed	Explain that the therapeutic effect will be delayed
Anticoagulants (Coumadin and others)	Food high in vitamin K: citrus fruits, egg yolks, large amounts of fish, fish oil, potato chips, vegetable oil, leafy green vegetables	Decrease prothrombin time	Watch for changes in prothrombin time, limit intake of foods high in vitamin K
Bisacodyl tablets	Milk or alkalinizing food	Disintegrate the enteric coating prematurely in the stomach or intestine	Give the medication with water or another beverage. Watch for gastric irritation or lack of therapeutic effect if the patient did take milk
Cardiac glycosides	Milk or other food high in calcium	Diminish the therapeutic effect and lead to arrhythmia	Withhold milk; give the drug after meals to lessen gastric irritation
Erythromycin stearate	Acidic fruit or juice, carbonated beverages	Decompose the drug prematurely	Give the drug 1 hour before or 3 hours after meals
Griseofulvin	Very little fat	Cause incomplete absorption of the drug	Serve butter or margarine at each meal
Iron salts	Cereal, eggs, milk	Form insoluble chelates	Withhold these foods

If your patient takes:	And eats or drinks:	The combination may:	So intervene to:
Iron salts	Citrus fruit juice	Hasten absorption and cause toxic reactions: nausea, vomiting, peripheral vascular collapse, anaphylaxis	Withhold these juices
Levodopa (Larodopa, Sinemet)	Foods high in vitamin B₆— yeast, liver, muscle meat, whole grain cereals, fish, vegetables, molasses	Interfere with the therapeutic effect	Limit intake of these foods
Lincomycin (Lincocin)	Any food or beverage	Interfere with absorption of the drug	Allow only water for 1-2 hours before and after administration of the drug
Lithium	Insufficient salt and water	Cause lithium toxicity: diarrhea, vomiting, drowsiness, muscular weakness, lack of coordination	Insure adequate salt and fluid intake; watch for toxicity
MAO inhibitors	Foods high in pressor amines: aged cheese, processed cheese, beer, wine (especially Chianti), chocolate, yeast extract, avocado, pickled herring, chicken liver, broad bean pods	Cause possibly fatal hypertensive crisis or intracranial bleeding	Warn patients of the danger; watch for signs of crisis: severe headache, chest pain, profuse sweating, palpitation, fast or slow pulse, visual disturbances, stertorous breathing, coma

Foods that foil drugs
(continued)

If your patient takes:	And eats or drinks:	The combination may:	So intervene to:
Penicillin	Acidic fruit juices or beverages	Decompose the drug prematurely	Give the drug with water on an empty stomach
Tetrachloroethylene (anthelmintic therapy)	Excessive fat	Cause systemic absorption and CNS toxicity instead of topical action	Restrict fat intake
Tetracycline antibiotics	Any food, but especially milk and other dairy products	Interfere with absorption of the drug	Give the drug 1 hour before or 2 hours after meals
Thiazide diuretics	Imported (natural extract) licorice	Cause hypokalemia, salt and water retention, hypertension, alkalosis	Warn the patient to avoid imported licorice; most domestic licorice contains only harmless artificial flavoring
Tolbutamide	Alcohol	Cause photosensitivity and disulfiramlike reactions	Warn the patient to avoid alcoholic beverages

ish the effectiveness of one of the drugs. And this can lead to the failure of therapy of the disease that the drug is intended to control. It is difficult to judge what a drug combination will do in a patient, since the same combination of drugs may act differently in individual patients.

More than half of elderly patients use a prescription drug and an OTC remedy or alcohol at the same time (a surprising number of OTC formulations contain alcohol, some up to 42 per cent!). Use of laxatives is particularly widespread among the elderly, and is the cause of unwanted effects with regard to drug absorption.

Clearly, physicians must query their older patients on their total drug diet, prescribed and OTC. And they should question them often on this matter. Physicians and pharmacists should counsel the elderly on what foods and OTC drugs can cause problems when mixed with prescription medications (see the accompanying "Foods that foil drugs") and whether alcohol interacts with any one of them. The pharmacist is in a position to maintain patients' drug profiles and monitor them for any combinations that could cause unfavorable interactions. Surrounded by virtually all nonprescription formulations available, in many cases he can observe which OTC drugs his elderly customers are in the habit of buying. He is in a position also to watch for any inappropriate prescribing on the part of physicians.

Altering the method of administration of a medicine can lead to undesired effects. Patients who have difficulty swallowing may crush tablets or open capsules and take the medication with a fluid or mixed with food. The change may affect absorption. See the accompanying list of drugs that shows whether a liquid form of a medication is available and whether a tablet can be crushed or a capsule opened without altering its effect.

The best approach to the danger of adverse reactions and drug-drug interactions is to cut down on their chances of occurring in the first place. Physicians caring for patients with several disorders should treat these disorders, so far as they can, one at a time. They should prescribe minimal doses and gradually build to the therapeutic dose, so they can monitor for adverse reactions. They should prescribe for a short period, and have refills cleared through them, so their patients' charts can be complete, up to date, and reliable for monitoring. Finally, physicians should know whether their patients' liver and kidney functions can successfully excrete the drugs, so that toxic levels do not build up.

Physicians and pharmacists should make sure their patients know the names of the medications they are taking. In case of an emergency, if the patient can tell the medical personnel what drugs he is taking and if the emergency condition is the result of overdose or failure of therapy, they will know what they are treating. They can also avoid medication that would interact with what the patient has been taking.

Patient noncompliance

The final step in the drug therapy of an illness is the patient's. Accurate diagnosis and appropriate prescribing don't cure or control a disease condition. That's accomplished only if the patient takes the medication in the right dosage at the right time.

But, often, this doesn't happen. Some patients forget a great deal of what their doctors tell them, and many, even if they do remember, don't understand the instructions. The problem in cases of misunderstanding doesn't always lie with the patient. Sometimes, physicians' prescribing is unclear. For example, if the instructions are no more explicit than to say "at mealtime," and if the patient ordinarily eats only two meals a day, he may take one fewer dose than the doctor intends. Some medications are to be taken on an empty stomach. Yet, if a prescription for one of them reads simply "three times a day," the patient is likely to interpret that as "at mealtime," and miss the therapeutic effect of the drug because it's not well absorbed.

Most problems of noncompliance, however, originate with the patients. The first remedy is education. There are seven points to cover when instructing elderly patients about a drug regimen:

• Patients should know what their pills are for. They can easily understand terms such as "blood pressure pill," "heart pill," and the like. If they know what their pills are for, they'll place greater importance on them, and have a greater sense of participating in their therapy—both of which will foster compliance.

• The patient should be able to repeat the correct dosage schedule and methods of administration for his medications and be given a chance to comment on whether these are realistic in terms of his daily routine.

• The patient should get a list of foods and drugs that may interact with the prescribed drugs and cause unwanted effects.

● It would increase compliance if the patient knew ahead of time when he should begin to feel a drug's therapeutic effect and also what side effects are likely. He should be encouraged to get in touch with the doctor if he finds the side effects are intolerable. The doctor can then assess the significance of the complaints and adjust the dosage or otherwise maintain therapy.

● Knowing how long the drug therapy is supposed to last would help compliance. Patients may discontinue drugs as soon as they feel better, and thereby increase chances for relapse or risk exacerbation of the illnesses. They should know why they must continue a medication and what they should do if they forget a dose.

● They should know, too, how long a prescription is supposed to last. Knowing when they are to get it refilled and seeing whether any pills are left at that time should indicate to them that they are not taking the medication as prescribed.

● It's also important to know how the drug is to be stored. Many drugs, to retain potency, require protection from light and must be kept in dark bottles. A drug can lose potency, too, beyond a length of time. If this is a factor for the type of drug the patient is to take, he should know what the expiration date is.

(Continued on page 132)

Crushing tablets, opening capsules: When is it safe?

Henry A. Palmer, Ph.D., and Gilles L. Fraser, R.Ph.

Swallowing a tablet or capsule ought to be simple, but it can be a difficult undertaking for the elderly. Most of the time these patients—or those who take care of them—can resort to the traditional solution of crushing the tablet or opening the capsule and mixing the medication with fluid or food. But some drugs now come in forms that can't be altered without changing therapeutic effect. Among the noncrushable forms are enteric coated tablets, designed for dissolution in the intestine rather than in the stomach; tablets coated to give both immediate and delayed action; tablets within tablets, usually of different colors, for the same purpose; uncoated tablets speckled with beads for delayed action; uncoated tablets designed to dissolve in the mouth for absorption through the oral mucosa. Capsules containing beads or pellets, usually for delayed action, may be opened and the contents ingested, but only if they are not crushed or chewed. But since this is difficult to assure, it's better not to open these capsules.

Even if a tablet can be crushed safely, a liquid formulation of the drug may be available. But remember that liquid formulations dissolve quickly into the bloodstream, so they can't take the place of prolonged-release tablets.

The following table lists 190 common oral drugs or combination products, and tells whether a liquid formulation is available and whether you can safely crush the tablet or open the capsule.

Product	Solid formulation	Liquid formulation	May tablet be crushed or capsule opened?
Achromycin (tetracycline)	100-, 250-, 500-mg capsules	125 mg/5 ml	Yes
Actifed	Tablet with 2.5 mg triprolidine, 60 mg pseudoephedrine	1.25 mg triprolidine, 30 mg pseudoephedrine/5 ml	Yes
Adapin (doxepin)	10-, 25-, 50-, 100-mg capsules	None	Yes
Aldactazide	Tablet with 25 mg hydrochlorothiazide, 25 mg spironolactone	None	Yes
Aldactone (spironolactone)	25-mg tablet	None	Yes
Aldomet (methyldopa)	125-, 250-, 500-mg tablets	None	Yes
Aldoril	Tablets with 15 or 25 mg hydrochlorothiazide, 250 mg methyldopa; 30 or 50 mg hydrochlorothiazide, 500 mg methyldopa	None	Yes
Amcill (ampicillin)	250-, 500-mg capsules; 125-mg chewable tablet	125 mg/5 ml, 250 mg/5 ml	Yes

Crushing tablets, opening capsules: When is it safe? (continued)

Product	Solid formulation	Liquid formulation	May tablet be crushed or capsule opened?
Amoxil (amoxicillin)	250-, 500-mg capsules	125 mg/5 ml, 250 mg/5 ml	Yes
Antivert (meclizine)	12.5-, 25-mg tablets; 25-mg chewable tablet	None	Yes
Apresoline (hydralazine)	10-, 25-, 50-, 100-mg tablets	None	Yes
Aristocort (triamcinolone)	1-, 2-, 4-, 8-, 16-mg tablets	2 mg/5 ml	Yes
Artane (trihexyphenidyl)	2-, 5-mg tablets 5-mg sustained-release capsule	2 mg/5 ml	Yes (tablets) No (capsule)
Atarax (hydroxyzine)	10-, 25-, 50-, 100-mg tablets	10 mg/5 ml	Yes
Ativan (lorazepam)	0.5-, 1-, 2-mg tablets	None	Yes
Atromid-S (clofibrate)	500-mg capsule	None	Yes*

*It may be difficult to extract the contents of the capsule completely.

Product	Solid formulation	Liquid formulation	May tablet be crushed or capsule opened?
Aventyl (nortriptyline)	10-, 25-mg capsules	10 mg/5 ml	Yes
Azo Gantrisin	Tablet with 500 mg sulfisoxazole, 50 mg phenazopyridine	None	Yes*
Bactrim	Tablets with 400 mg sulfamethoxazole, 80 mg trimethoprim; 800 mg sulfamethoxazole, 160 mg trimethoprim	200 mg sulfamethoxazole, 40 mg trimethoprim/5 ml	Yes
Benadryl (diphenhydramine)	25-, 50-mg capsules	12.5 mg/5 ml	Yes
Bentyl (dicyclomine)	10-mg capsule, 20-mg tablet	10 mg/5 ml	Yes
Bentyl with phenobarbital	Capsule with 10 mg dicyclomine, 15 mg phenobarbital; tablet with 20 mg dicyclomine, 15 mg phenobarbital	10 mg dicyclomine, 15 mg phenobarbital/5 ml	Yes
Brethine (terbutaline)	2.5-, 5-mg tablets	None	Yes

*May stain teeth if crushed tablet is in prolonged contact with them.

Crushing tablets, opening capsules: When is it safe? (continued)

Product	Solid formulation	Liquid formulation	May tablet be crushed or capsule opened?
Butazolidin Alka	Capsule with 100 mg phenylbutazone, 100 mg aluminum hydroxide, 150 mg magnesium trisilicate	None	Yes
Butisol Sodium (butabarbital)	15-, 30-, 50-, 100-mg tablets and capsules	30 mg/5 ml	Yes
Cardilate (erythrityl tetranitrate)	5-, 10-, 15-mg tablets; 10-mg chewable tablet	None	Yes
Catapres (clonidine)	0.1-, 0.2-mg tablets	None	Yes
Cedilanid (lanatoside C)	0.5-mg tablet	None	Yes
Chlor-Trimeton (chlorpheniramine)	4-mg tablet; 8-, 12-mg repeat-action tablets	2 mg/5 ml	Yes (4-mg tablet) No (repeat-action tablets)
Cleocin (clindamycin)	75-, 150-mg capsules	75 mg/5 ml	Yes

Product	Solid formulation	Liquid formulation	May tablet be crushed or capsule opened?
Cogentin (benztropine mesylate)	0.5-, 1-, 2-mg tablets	None	Yes
Combid	Sustained-action capsule with 5 mg isopropamide, 10 mg prochlorperazine	None	No
Compazine (prochlorperazine)	5-, 10-, 25-mg tablets; 10-, 15-, 30-, 75-mg sustained-action capsules	5 mg/5 ml, 10 mg/ml	Yes (tablets) No (capsules)
Coumadin (warfarin)	2-, 2.5-, 5-, 7.5-, 10-mg tablets	None	Yes
Cyclospasmol (cyclandelate)	100-mg tablet; 200-, 400-mg capsules	None	Yes
Dalmane (flurazepam)	15-, 30-mg capsules	None	Yes
Darvon (propoxyphene)	32-, 65-mg capsules	None	Yes
Daxolin (loxapine)	10-, 25-, 50-mg capsules	25 mg/ml	Yes

Crushing tablets, opening capsules:
When is it safe? (continued)

Product	Solid formulation	Liquid formulation	May tablet be crushed or capsule opened?
Demerol (meperidine)	50-, 100-mg tablets	50 mg/5 ml	Yes
Desoxyn (methamphetamine)	2.5-, 5-mg tablets; 5-, 10-, 15-mg sustained-release tablets	None	Yes (plain tablets) No (sustained-release tablets)
Diabinese (chlorpropamide)	100-, 250-mg tablets	None	Yes
Diamox (acetazolamide)	125-, 250-mg tablets 500-mg sustained-action capsule	None	Yes (tablets) No (capsule)
Dilantin	30-, 100-mg capsules (phenytoin sodium)	30 mg/5 ml, 125 mg/5 ml (phenytoin)	Yes
Dimetapp	Sustained-release tablet with 12 mg brompheniramine, 15 mg phenylephrine, 15 mg phenylpropanolamine	4 mg brompheniramine, 5 mg phenylephrine, 5 mg phenylpropanolamine/5 ml	No
Diupres	Tablet with 250 or 500 mg chlorothiazide, 0.125 mg reserpine	None	Yes
Diuril (chlorothiazide)	250-, 500-mg tablets	250 mg/5 ml	Yes

Product	Solid formulation	Liquid formulation	May tablet be crushed or capsule opened?
Donnatal	Tablet and capsule with 16.2 mg phenobarbital, 0.1037 mg hyoscyamine sulfate, 0.0194 mg atropine sulfate, 0.0065 mg hyoscine hydrobromide	Identical combination in 5 ml elixir	Yes
Donnatal Extentabs	Sustained-action tablet with 48.6 mg phenobarbital, 0.3111 mg hyoscyamine sulfate, 0.0582 mg atropine sulfate, 0.0195 mg hyoscine hydrobromide	None	No
Doriden (glutethimide)	500-mg capsule; 250-, 500-mg tablets	None	Yes
Dyazide	Capsule with 50 mg triamterene, 25 mg hydrochlorothiazide	None	Yes
Dyrenium (triamterene)	50-, 100-mg capsules	None	Yes
Edecrin (ethacrynic acid)	25-, 50-mg tablets	None	Yes

Crushing tablets, opening capsules: When is it safe? (continued)

Product	Solid formulation	Liquid formulation	May tablet be crushed or capsule opened?
Elavil (amitriptyline)	10-, 25-, 50-, 75-, 100-, 150-mg tablets	None	Yes
Elixophyllin (theophylline)	100-, 200-mg capsules 125-, 250-mg sustained-release capsules	80 mg/15 ml	Yes (plain capsules) No (sustained-release capsules)
Empirin Compound/Codeine	Tablet with 227 mg aspirin, 162 mg phenacetin, 32 mg caffeine, and codeine in one of the following strengths: 7.5, 15, 30, 60 mg	None	Yes
E-Mycin (erythromycin)	250-mg enteric-coated tablet	None	No
Enduron (methyclothiazide)	2.5-, 5-mg tablets	None	Yes
Equagesic	Tablet with 150 mg meprobamate, 75 mg ethoheptazine, 250 mg aspirin	None	Yes

Product	Solid formulation	Liquid formulation	May tablet be crushed or capsule opened?
Equanil (meprobamate)	200-, 400-mg tablets 400-mg capsule	None	Yes
Erythrocin (erythromycin stearate)	125-, 250-, 500-mg tablets	None	No
Esidrix (hydrochlorothiazide)	25-, 50-, 100-mg tablets	None	Yes
Etrafon	Tablets with 10 mg amitriptyline, 2 mg perphenazine; 10 mg amitriptyline, 4 mg perphenazine; 25 mg amitriptyline, 2 mg perphenazine; 25 mg amitriptyline, 4 mg perphenazine	None	Yes
Feosol (ferrous sulfate)	325 mg tablet 250-mg capsule	220 mg/5 ml	No
Fiorinal	Tablet and capsule with 50 mg butalbital, 40 mg caffeine, 200 mg aspirin, 130 mg phenacetin	None	Yes

Crushing tablets, opening capsules: When is it safe? (continued)

Product	Solid formulation	Liquid formulation	May tablet be crushed or capsule opened?
Flagyl (metronidazole)	250-mg tablet	None	Yes
Flexeril (cyclobenzaprine)	10-mg tablet	None	Yes
Gantanol (sulfamethoxazole)	500-mg, 1-gm tablets	500 mg/5 ml	Yes
Gantrisin (sulfisoxazole)	500-mg tablet	500 mg/5 ml, 1 gm/5 ml	Yes
Haldol (haloperidol)	0.5-, 1-, 2-, 5-, 10-mg tablets	2 mg/ml	Yes
Hydergine	1-mg tablet; 0.5-, 1-mg sublingual tablets	None	Yes (1-mg tablet) No (sublingual tablets)
HydroDIURIL (hydrochlorothiazide)	25-, 50-, 100-mg tablets	None	Yes

Product	Solid formulation	Liquid formulation	May tablet be crushed or capsule opened?
Hydromox (quinethazone)	50-mg tablet	None	Yes
Hydropres	Tablets with 25 or 50 mg hydrochlorothiazide, 0.125 mg reserpine	None	Yes
Hygroton (chlorthalidone)	25-, 50-, 100-mg tablets	None	Yes
Ilosone (erythromycin)	125-, 250-mg capsules; 500-mg tablet; 125-, 250-mg chewable tablets	125 mg/5 ml, 250 mg/5 ml, 100 mg/ml	Yes
Inderal (propranolol)	10-, 20-, 40-, 80-mg tablets	None	Yes
Indocin (indomethacin)	25-, 50-mg capsules	None	Yes
Ionamin (phentermine)	15-, 30-mg capsules	None	No
Ismelin (guanethidine)	10-, 25-mg tablets	None	Yes

Crushing tablets, opening capsules:
When is it safe? (continued)

Product	Solid formulation	Liquid formulation	May tablet be crushed or capsule opened?
Isordil (isosorbide)	10-mg chewable tablet; 5-, 10-, 20-mg tablets; 40-mg sustained-action tablet and capsule; 2.5-, 5-mg sublingual tablets; 40-mg sustained-release capsule and tablet	None	Yes (plain and chewable tablets) No (other forms)
Kantrex (kanamycin)	500-mg capsule	None	Yes
Keflex (cephalexin)	250-, 500-mg capsules, 1-gm tablet	125 mg/5 ml, 250 mg/5 ml	Yes
Lanoxin (digoxin)	0.125-, 0.25-, 0.5-mg tablets	0.05 mg/ml	Yes
Larodopa (levodopa)	100-, 250-, 500-mg tablets and capsules	None	Yes
Larotid (amoxicillin)	250-, 500-mg capsules	125 mg/5 ml, 250 mg/5 ml	Yes
Lasix (furosemide)	20-, 40-mg tablets	10 mg/ml	Yes

Product	Solid formulation	Liquid formulation	May tablet be crushed or capsule opened?
Librax	Capsule with 2.5 mg clidinium, 5 mg chlordiazepoxide	None	Yes
Librium (chlordiazepoxide)	5-, 10-, 25-mg capsules	None	Yes
Lidone (molindone)	5-, 10-, 25-mg capsules	None	Yes
Lincocin (lincomycin)	500-mg capsule	250 mg/5 ml	Yes
Lomotil	Tablet with 2.5 mg diphenoxylate, 0.025 mg atropine sulfate	Identical combination in 5 ml liquid	Yes
Loxitane (loxapine)	5-, 10-, 25-, 50-mg capsules	25 mg/ml	Yes
Macrodantin (nitrofurantoin)	25-, 50-, 100-mg capsules	Furadantin 25 mg/5 ml	Yes
Marax	Tablet with 130 mg theophylline, 25 mg ephedrine, 10 mg hydroxyzine	32.5 mg theophylline, 6.25 mg ephedrine, 2.5 mg hydroxyzine/5 ml	Yes

Crushing tablets, opening capsules: When is it safe? (continued)

Product	Solid formulation	Liquid formulation	May tablet be crushed or capsule opened?
Medrol (methylprednisolone)	2-, 4-, 8-, 16-, 24-, 32-mg tablets	None	No
Mellaril (thioridazine)	10-, 15-, 25-, 50-, 100-, 150-, 200-mg tablets	30 mg/ml, 100 mg/ml	Yes
Mephyton (phytonadione)	5-mg tablet	None	Yes
Minocin (minocycline)	50-, 100-mg capsules	50 mg/5 ml	Yes
Moban (molindone)	5-, 10-, 25-mg tablets	None	Yes
Motrin (ibuprofen)	300-, 400-mg tablets	None	Yes
Mysoline (primidone)	50-, 250-mg tablets	250 mg/5 ml	Yes
Naprosyn (naproxen)	250-mg tablet	None	Yes

Product	Solid formulation	Liquid formulation	May tablet be crushed or capsule opened?
Nardil (phenelzine)	15-mg tablet	None	Yes
Navane (thiothixene)	1-, 2-, 5-, 10-, 20-mg capsules	5 mg/ml	Yes
NegGram (nalidixic acid)	250-, 500-mg, 1-gm tablets	250 mg/5 ml	Yes
Nembutal (pentobarbital)	30-, 50-, 100-mg capsules	18.2 mg/5 ml	Yes
Nicolar (niacin)	500-mg tablet	None	Yes
Nitro-Bid (nitroglycerin for oral administration)	2.5-, 6.5-, 9-mg capsules	None	No
Noludar (methyprylon)	50-, 200-mg tablets; 300-mg capsule	None	Yes

Crushing tablets, opening capsules: When is it safe? (continued)

Product	Solid formulation	Liquid formulation	May tablet be crushed or capsule opened?
Norgesic	Tablets with 225 mg aspirin, 160 mg phenacetin, 30 mg caffeine, 25 mg orphenadrine; 450 mg aspirin, 320 mg phenacetin, 60 mg caffeine, 50 mg orphenadrine	None	Yes
Norpramin (desipramine)	25-, 50-, 75-, 100-, 150-mg tablets	None	Yes
Omnipen (ampicillin)	250-, 500-mg capsules	125 mg/5 ml, 250 mg/5 ml, 500 mg/5 ml	Yes
Orinase (tolbutamide)	500-mg tablet	None	Yes
Ornade	Sustained-action capsule with 50 mg phenylpropanolamine, 8 mg chlorpheniramine, 2.5 mg isopropamide	None	No
Oxalid (oxyphenbutazone)	100-mg tablet	None	Yes
Pamelor (nortriptyline)	10-, 25-mg capsules	10 mg/5 ml	Yes

Product	Solid formulation	Liquid formulation	May tablet be crushed or capsule opened?
Parafon Forte	Tablet with 300 mg acetaminophen, 250 mg chlorzoxazone	None	Yes
Parnate (tranylcypromine)	10-mg tablet	None	Yes
Pavabid (papaverine)	150-, 300-mg capsules	None	No
SK-Penicillin VK (penicillin V)	250-, 500-mg tablets	125 mg/5 ml, 250 mg/5 ml	Yes
Pentids (penicillin G)	200,000 U (125 mg), 400,000 U (250 mg), 800,000 U (500 mg) tablets	200,000 U (125 mg)/5 ml, 400,000 U (250 mg)/5 ml	Yes
Percodan	Tablet with 224 mg aspirin, 160 mg phenacetin, 32 mg caffeine, and 4.5 or 2.25 mg oxycodone hydrochloride and 0.38 or 0.19 mg oxycodone terephthalate	None	Yes
Periactin (cyproheptadine)	4-mg tablet	2 mg/5 ml	Yes

Crushing tablets, opening capsules:
When is it safe? (continued)

Product	Solid formulation	Liquid formulation	May tablet be crushed or capsule opened?
Permitil (fluphenazine)	0.25-, 2.5-, 5-, 10-mg tablets; 1-mg repeat-action tablet	5 mg/ml	Yes (plain tablets) No (repeat-action tablet)
Pertofrane (desipramine)	25-, 50-mg capsules	None	Yes
Phenaphen/Codeine	Tablets with 325 mg acetaminophen, and codeine in one of the following strengths: 15, 30, or 60 mg; 650 mg acetaminophen, 30 mg codeine	None	Yes
Phenergan (promethazine)	12.5-, 25-, 50-mg tablets	6.25 mg/5 ml, 25 mg/5 ml	Yes
Phenobarbital	15-, 30-, 65-, 100-mg tablets	20 mg/5 ml	Yes
Placidyl (ethchlorvynol)	100-, 200-, 500-, 750-mg capsules	None	Yes
Polaramine (dexchlorpheniramine)	4-, 6-mg repeat-action tablets	2 mg/5 ml	No

Product	Solid formulation	Liquid formulation	May tablet be crushed or capsule opened?
Polycillin (ampicillin)	250-, 500-mg capsules	125 mg/5 ml, 250 mg/5 ml, 500 mg/5 ml	Yes
Prednisone	2.5-, 5-, 10-, 20-, 50-mg tablets	None	Yes
Premarin (conjugated estrogen)	0.3-, 0.625-, 1.25, 2.5-mg tablets	None	Yes
Principen (ampicillin)	250-, 500-mg capsules	125 mg/5 ml, 250 mg/5 ml	Yes
Pro-Banthine (propantheline)	7.5-, 15-mg tablets, 30-mg sustained-release tablet	None	Yes (plain tablets) No (sustained-release tablet)
Prolixin (fluphenazine)	1-, 2.5-, 5-, 10-mg tablets	2.5 mg/5 ml	Yes
Proloid (thyroid globulin)	¼-, ½-, 1-, 1½-, 2-, 3-, 5-gr tablets	None	Yes
Pronestyl (procainamide)	250-, 375-, 500-mg tablets and capsules	None	Yes

Crushing tablets, opening capsules:
When is it safe? (continued)

Product	Solid formulation	Liquid formulation	May tablet be crushed or capsule opened?
Provera (medroxyprogesterone)	2.5-, 10-mg tablets	None	Yes
Pyridium (phenazopyridine)	100-, 200-mg tablets	None	No
Quibron	Capsules with 150 mg theophylline, 90 mg guaifenesin; 300 mg theophylline, 180 mg guaifenesin	150 mg theophylline, 90 mg guaifenesin/15 ml	Yes
Regroton	Capsule with 25 mg chlorthalidone, 0.125 mg reserpine; 50 mg chlorthalidone, 0.25 mg reserpine	None	Yes
Renese (polythiazide)	1-, 2-, 4-mg tablets	None	Yes
Rifadin (rifampin)	300-mg capsule	None	Yes
Ritalin (methylphenidate)	5-, 10-, 20-mg tablets	None	Yes

Product	Solid formulation	Liquid formulation	May tablet be crushed or capsule opened?
Robitet (tetracycline)	250-, 500-mg capsules	125 mg/5 ml	Yes
Salutensin	Tablets with 25 or 50 mg hydroflumethiazide, 0.125 reserpine	None	Yes
Septra	Tablets with 400 mg sulfamethoxazole, 80 mg trimethoprim; 800 mg sulfamethoxazole, 160 mg trimethoprim	200 mg sulfamethoxazole, 40 mg trimethoprim/5 ml	Yes
Serax (oxazepam)	10-, 15-, 30-mg capsules 15-mg tablet	None	Yes
Serentil (mesoridazine besylate)	10-, 25-, 50, 100-mg tablets	25 mg/ml	Yes
Sinemet	Tablets with 10 mg carbidopa, 100 mg levodopa; 25 mg carbidopa, 250 mg levodopa	None	Yes
Sinequan (doxepin)	10-, 25-, 50-, 75-, 100-, 150-mg capsules	10 mg/ml	Yes
Singlet	Tablet with 40 mg phenylephrine, 8 mg chlorpheniramine, 500 mg acetaminophen	None	No

Crushing tablets, opening capsules: When is it safe? (continued)

Product	Solid formulation	Liquid formulation	May tablet be crushed or capsule opened?
Slo-Phyllin (theophylline)	100-, 200-mg tablets; 60-, 125-, 250-mg timed-release capsules	80 mg/15 ml	No
Slow-K (potassium chloride)	600-mg slow-release tablet	None	No
Sorbitrate (isosorbide)	5-, 10-, 20-mg tablets; 5-, 10-mg chewable tablets; 40-mg sustained-action tablet; 2.5-, 5-mg sublingual tablets	None	Yes (plain and chewable tablets) No (other forms)
Stelazine (trifluoperazine)	1-, 2-, 5-, 10-mg tablets	10 mg/ml	Yes
Sudafed (pseudoephedrine)	30-, 60-mg tablets	30 mg/5 ml	Yes
Suladyne	Tablet with 125 mg sulfamethizole, 125 mg sulfadiazine, 75 mg phenazopyridine	None	Yes*
Sumycin (tetracycline)	250-, 500-mg tablets and capsules	125 mg/5 ml	Yes

*May stain teeth if crushed tablet is in prolonged contact with them.

Product	Solid formulation	Liquid formulation	May tablet be crushed or capsule opened?
Symmetrel (amantadine)	100-mg capsule	50 mg/5 ml	Yes
Synalgos-DC	Capsule with 194.4 mg aspirin, 162 mg phenacetin, 30 mg caffeine, 16 mg dihydrocodeine, 6.25 mg promethazine	None	Yes
Synthroid (levothyroxine)	0.025-, 0.05-, 0.1-, 0.15-, 0.2-, 0.3-mg tablets	None	Yes
Tagamet (cimetidine)	300-mg tablet	None	Yes
Talwin (pentazocine)	50-mg tablet	None	Yes
Tandearil (oxyphenbutazone)	100-mg tablet	None	Yes
Taractan (chlorprothixene)	10-, 25-, 50, 100-mg tablets	100 mg/5 ml	Yes

Crushing tablets, opening capsules: When is it safe? (continued)

Product	Solid formulation	Liquid formulation	May tablet be crushed or capsule opened?
Tedral	Tablet with 130 mg theophylline, 24 mg ephedrine, 8 mg phenobarbital	65 mg theophylline, 12 mg ephedrine, 4 mg phenobarbital/5 ml (suspension); 32.5 mg theophylline, 6 mg ephedrine, 2 mg phenobarbital/5 ml (elixir)	Yes
Teldrin (chlorpheniramine)	8-, 12-mg sustained-action capsules	None	No
Tenuate (diethylpropion)	25-, 75-mg tablets	None	No
Thorazine (chlorpromazine)	10-, 25-, 50-, 100-, 200-mg tablets; 30-, 75-, 150-, 200-mg sustained-action capsules	10 mg/5 ml, 30 mg/ml, 100 mg/ml	Yes (tablets) No (capsules)
Tigan (trimethobenzamide)	100-, 250-mg capsules	None	Yes
Tofranil (imipramine)	10-, 25-, 50-mg tablets	None	Yes
Tolectin (tolmetin sodium)	500-mg tablet	None	Yes

Product	Solid formulation	Liquid formulation	May tablet be crushed or capsule opened?
Tolinase (tolazamide)	100-, 250-, 500-mg tablets	None	Yes
Tranxene (clorazepate)	3.75-, 7.5-, 15-mg capsules 11.25, 22.5 mg single-dose tablets	None	Yes (capsules) No (tablets)
Tremin (trihexyphenidyl)	2-, 5-mg tablets	None	Yes
Triavil	Tablets with 10 mg amitriptyline, 2 mg perphenazine; 10 mg amitriptyline, 4 mg perphenazine; 25 mg amitriptyline, 2 mg perphenazine; 25 mg amitriptyline, 4 mg perphenazine; 50 mg amitriptyline, 4 mg perphenazine	None	Yes
Triclos (triclofos)	75-mg tablet	100 mg/ml	Yes
Tylenol (acetaminophen)	325-, 500-mg tablet, 80-mg chewable tablet, 500-mg capsule	60 mg/0.6 ml, 120 mg/5 ml, 1000 mg/30 ml	Yes

Crushing tablets, opening capsules: When is it safe? (continued)

Product	Solid formulation	Liquid formulation	May tablet be crushed or capsule opened?
Valium (diazepam)	2-, 5-, 10-mg tablets	None	Yes
Vasodilan (isoxsuprine)	10-, 20-mg tablets	None	Yes
V-Cillin K (penicillin)	125-, 250-, 500-mg tablets	125 mg/5 ml, 250 mg/5 ml	Yes
Verstran (prazepam)	10-mg tablet	None	Yes
Vesprin (triflupromazine)	10-, 25-, 50-mg tablets	50 mg/5 ml	Yes
Vibramycin (doxycycline)	50-, 100-mg capsules	25 mg/5 ml, 50 mg/5 ml	Yes
Vistaril (hydroxyzine)	25-, 50-, 100-mg capsules	25 mg/5 ml	Yes

Product	Solid formulation	Liquid formulation	May tablet be crushed or capsule opened?
Vivactil (protriptyline)	5-, 10-mg tablets	None	Yes
Zaroxolyn (metolazone)	2.5-, 5-, 10-mg tablets	None	Yes
Zyloprim (allopurinol)	100-, 300-mg tablets	None	Yes

Pharmacists who keep patients' drug profiles can tell when a patient is due to come in for a refill of a medication for a chronic condition. If the patient fails to come in on time, this could be an indication that he's skipping some dose—and this can exacerbate a chronic condition. Coming in too soon can mean the patient is taking too many pills and is running a risk of drug toxicity.

Besides education, there are other remedies to overcome obstacles to compliance. One of the first problems is the cap on the medication bottle. Child-proof caps are impossible for many elderly to remove, and if they live alone, they may be unable to take the medication. It would be a simple matter for a physician's office to have a supply of typical child-proof containers on hand. The physician or one of his assistants can take an elderly patient through a trial to see if the patient is able to manipulate the caps. Any patient who cannot open a bottle should be told to specify regular caps when getting prescriptions filled and refilled. The physician may specify regular caps on the prescription.

The elderly with failing vision may have difficulty reading labels for dosage information and even distinguishing one bottle of pills from another. One remedy is to have labels typed in large print and red ink. Similarly, they may find it hard to distinguish between pills. A patient on several drugs, all in the form of small, white tablets, may be very confused about which is which. The physician should prescribe the several drugs in different forms, if they're available, or even prescribe a drug from a different manufacturer in order to get a pill that is colored differently from the other drugs the patient is taking. A pill readily distinguishable from others is more likely to be taken correctly.

Memory aids are easy to propose and create, and in view of the improved compliance and consequent improved health of the patient, they're worth the effort. One simple device the physician's office staff can prepare for elderly patients who must take a number of pills is a chart that outlines information about the drugs and instructions for taking them. The information should include the names of the drugs, what they're for (e.g., "heart pill"), and when they should be taken. Sample pills can be taped to the chart to aid in identification.

Originally suggested in the July 1977 *Hospital Physician* as an aid for pediatric patients who have complex drug regimens, "the medicine box" can be used as well with geriatric patients who require many medications. The medicine box is a set of 28 dark-colored vials,

A prescriber's checklist

When deciding on a drug program for an elderly patient—or during a periodic review of such a program—you can use this list of questions to help you do your part in keeping your patient from making medication mistakes and from adverse reactions or drug interactions.

- Does this patient have impaired kidney or liver function? What's the route of excretion of the drug I'm prescribing?

- Does this patient really need all the medicines I've prescribed for him? Can he get along well enough without one or more of them?

- What is the smallest dose that still has adequate therapeutic effect?

- What other drugs—prescribed and OTC—does this patient take?

- Does this patient use laxatives?

- Does this patient drink?

- Does food have an effect on absorption of this drug? Does this patient eat three meals a day regularly? Does he go days without eating? Is any food known to interact with this drug?

- Is there any easy-to-administer form of the drug?

- Is there a family member or friend I can explain the drug regimen to and can count on to ensure compliance?

- Can the patient repeat to me the drug's name, what it's for, and the dosage instructions?
- Can the patient see well enough to read the label and to distinguish one kind of pill from another?
- Are my label instructions unambiguous?
- Can the patient manipulate a child-proof cap?
- What side effects should this patient expect? Has he ever complained about side effects? Have I ever asked him about side effects?
- Are there one-a-day strengths I can prescribe for nighttime use so the patient can sleep through the worst of the side effects?
- Does the patient know when to expect the therapeutic effect? How long is the patient's therapy to last?
- Can this patient afford the medicine? Does he need advice on financial aid programs he may be eligible for?
- Does the patient's chart show all the refills he's been getting?
- What memory aids are suitable for this patient?

arranged in a box in seven rows of four, one row for each day of the week. The cap of each vial in a row of four is labeled "morn," "noon," "eve," or "night." An entire week's supply of pills can be divided into doses, and the patient need go to only one vial for each drug administration. The proper daily doses are already meted out, and of course, a vial still with its pills is a clear indication that a dose is being missed.

Using the same principle, but on a smaller scale, one day's medications can be divided into vials that have caps colored differently for the times of the day the pills are to be taken, in a sequence that is easy to remember, such as red, white, and blue—with black for a fourth, nighttime dose, if required.

One reason patients fail to comply with a drug regimen is that they don't want to feel the side effects. If the medication that causes the disagreeable effects can be dispensed in a one-a-day strength, it can be taken at night, so the patient will sleep through the worst of the side effects. One-a-day medications that have sedative effects, if taken at bedtime, can improve sleep.

A problem with nighttime medication is the risk of overdose, especially with pills to aid sleep. A patient may awaken during the night and, in a half-awake state, not remember whether he took his bedtime pill. If he should take another, it may cause him to be groggy and confused into the next day. One easy way to prevent such an overdose is to have the patient make a point of placing the nighttime pill on his bedside table and keeping the bottle elsewhere. If he awakes and sees no pill on the table, he can be sure of having taken it.

Another method is to put a week's supply of nighttime pills in envelopes marked for each day of the week and to seal the envelopes. When the patient takes his dose, he leaves the opened envelope on the bedside table as a reminder that he has taken it.

Depression and loneliness frequently cause elderly patients to stop caring whether they live or die, and accordingly, they stop taking their pills. As a consequence, they become confused, weak, and even further unable to cope. Physicians, nurses, and pharmacists shouldn't lose sight of the beneficial effects their interest and attention can have on these patients. Feeling worthwhile—because someone is interested in them—they become more willing to comply. Feeling better then because of the therapeutic effect of the medications, they'll be even better able to manage their drug regimens successfully.

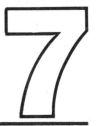

Nutrition in the Elderly: Practical Recommendations

By Myron Winick, M.D.

Nutrition is becoming increasingly important in the genesis of aging, the practical care of healthy old persons, and in the treatment of certain diseases of old age. Studies of the relationship, if any, between nutrition and longevity in animals showed that the life span of rats increased when the amount of food they ate during their first 20 days of life was restricted. And this increased life span was apparent even when the animals were weaned to a normal diet and allowed to eat whenever they wanted to for the rest of their lives.[1]

The effects of nutrition on longevity were even more dramatic when, after the rats were weaned, they were fed restricted amounts of a normal diet. Their life expectancy nearly doubled.[1] Some animals lived more than 1,800 days—equivalent to 180 years in man.

The longer life of these animals was related, in large measure, to a decrease in the incidence of certain diseases common to elderly rats. For example, glomerulonephrosis was rare in animals whose diets were chronically restricted, whereas as many as 40 per cent of full-fed rats developed this debilitating, age-dependent kidney disease. In addition, the incidence of such diseases as myocardial fibrosis, peribronchial lymphocytosis, periarteritis, prostatitis, and endocrine hyperplasias decreased by about 50 to 90 per cent. The relatively few cases that did occur were usually mild and they developed at a very old age.[1]

These animal experiments are important because they indicate that life can be prolonged before some of the common diseases of old age begin.

I've cited overall life expectancy data. However, the incidence of any *particular* age-related disease may not follow this pattern. Renal, myocardial, and prostatic disease increased in rats fed relatively high-protein diets. These findings suggest that the quantity as well as the quality of the diets fed is important in the aging process. However, we cannot yet make clinical recommendations based on these data.

Does the quality of the diet fed influence longevity? Only insofar as carbohydrate is concerned. Longevity seemed to be strongly related to the relative amount of carbohydrate the animals consumed. As it increased, life expectancy decreased.

However, diets were most effective when they were started during the first 5 to 10 per cent of the average life span for the species. If calories were restricted or dietary carbohydrate intake reduced at middle age, the animal's life expectancy *decreased*.[1] Thus, conditions for modifying longevity can be said to be age-dependent. But the animals must be young if dietary manipulation is to have the desired effect. Why and how diet affects longevity we can't say.

As clinicians we've learned the following from these experiments in animals:

1. Eating patterns set early in childhood can remain with an individual for many years, influencing the aging process.

2. Dietary manipulation from childhood through early adulthood is likely to affect the aging process.

3. Until data from studies in human populations become available, a moderate diet is a prudent approach—adequate calories for growth but not in excess.

4. Don't institute radical dietary changes late in life, except for a specific purpose. You're not likely to increase the individual's life span and may even decrease it.

Feeding the elderly

As aging progresses, cardiovascular, respiratory, and nervous system functions slowly but persistently deteriorate. From a nutritional standpoint, the most important age-related changes occur in the renal, neuromuscular, and gastrointestinal systems.

Under resting, steady-state conditions, most internal body organs continue to function fairly normally, even at advanced ages. Most functions decrease about 0.6 per cent per year throughout adult life.[2] However, kidney function clearly deteriorates with age, and gastrointestinal function declines.[2] Thus a number of processes basic to the digestion and absorption of nutrients are impaired, while others are unaffected. Among the processes affected by age are:

• Motor function. Muscle tone and strength decline with age. The weakening is probably caused by a decline in the number of functioning muscle fibers and in the contractile process itself.[2]

● Body composition. Almost everyone begins to lose skeletal bone by the time they're 50, but women tend to do so more than twice as rapidly as men. And we've always believed that as we grow older lean body mass is replaced by increased amounts of adipose tissue. This isn't true, according to recent data that suggest that lean body mass remains constant.[2] The implication is that lean body mass doesn't decline with age but that individuals with small, lean body masses tend to live longer. Also, adipocyte numbers actually increase very late in life, according to a series of recent studies in rats.[2]

We really don't know the significance of these findings, but they do suggest that old age is accompanied by relative obesity, probably caused by hyperplasia of adipose stores.[2]

These changes suggest that nutritional requirements for the elderly—especially specific nutrients—need to be evaluated. For example, the decrease in muscle mass with aging suggests that protein and amino acid requirements may change as one gets older. And as calcium absorption decreases and bone is resorbed, calcium and phosphorus requirements should also be re-evaluated. Iron and vitamin B_{12} requirements probably increase in the elderly, as their secretion of HCl decreases and the stomach atrophies.

Unfortunately, researchers are just beginning to study the nutritional requirements of the elderly. There are none for this age group, either in the current U.S. or international dietary allowances.

Protein and amino acids

Requirements for these nutrients don't seem to change with advancing age, even though the total daily amount of body protein synthesized declines.[3] It appears that the relative amounts of protein synthesized by various organs are redistributed. In the elderly, visceral tissue makes a greater contribution to total body protein synthesis, tempting one to predict that total protein requirements for the elderly are less per unit of body weight. But actual measurements of protein requirements by a variety of techniques suggest that the minimum protein needs of healthy adults do not change as they grow older. At present, the recommended intake for healthy men is 56 gm and for women, 46 gm. These amounts seem to be adequate for most healthy elderly persons.

As for amino acid requirements, those for threonine and tryptophan appear to be the same as for young adults, when expressed by unit of body weight, according to preliminary data. However, we know nothing about other amino acids.

Therefore, we can only base our decisions about protein and amino acid requirements for the elderly on very limited data. Under these circumstances, our decisions, at best, can only be educated guesses. Recognizing this, I'd recommend for the elderly a protein intake adequate to meet minimum daily requirements of a healthy young adult, but not much more. The protein should be rich in essential amino acids and supplied in an easily digested form—fish, soft cheese, lean meats, fowl, and certain vegetable proteins.

Nutritional supplements

As the elderly person's stomach may not be secreting adequate HCl, and intrinsic factor may be low, he or she may be prone to anemia. They may be unable to absorb adequate amounts of iron and vitamin B_{12}. Therefore, they need foods rich in these substances—red meat, liver, and fortified cereals. If they still develop anemia, then its specific cause must be determined and corrected. After that, supplements of iron and vitamin B_{12} are indicated.

Other vitamin and mineral requirements have not been worked out for the elderly. All you can do is provide them with the same amounts considered adequate for young adults. However, the elderly may be deficient in calcium.

Osteoporosis and periodontal disease

There are currently two schools of thought concerning the nature of osteoporosis and periodontal disease—two common, often debilitating diseases in older people. Some investigators believe the two are totally different diseases. Osteoporosis is considered a slowly progressing degenerative disease of bone, whereas periodontal disease is a chronic infection of the gums, with erosion of underlying bone. Others believe osteoporosis and periodontal disease are the same disease, caused by chronic, long-term calcium deficiency. Calcium is slowly drained from long bones and jaw bones so that individuals become susceptible to fractures of long bones. As bony sockets erode, teeth are lost.

My interpretation of the data leads me to believe that osteoporosis may be due, in part, to chronic calcium deficiency. Therefore, I would recommend foods rich in calcium throughout adult life as well as in childhood. For middle-aged patients with symptoms and X-ray findings of osteoporosis, 1 gm of calcium gluconate daily should be prescribed.

I'm not convinced that calcium supplements will prevent the disease from progressing, but risks associated with this form of prophylaxis are minimal, whereas the potential benefits are high enough to warrant the approach.

Data on periodontal disease are difficult to interpret. My feeling now is that it's a disease with multiple causes. Some forms may respond to calcium supplements, and I recommend them—again not because I'm convinced of their efficacy but because potential benefits outweigh risks.

Diseases common in the elderly

Certain diseases of the gastrointestinal tract are more common in the elderly, especially those who are affluent. These include diverticulitis, gallbladder disease, and cancer of the colon. Evidence suggests that all three may be related to the amount of fiber in the diet.

Diverticulitis becomes more prevalent as people grow older. But there are striking differences in its prevalence in developed Western countries compared with developing countries in the tropics. Yet, the incidence of diverticulitis does not correlate with the economic status of a country—it's low in Japan and Korea, for example. Genetic and racial factors seem to play a minor role—the disease is more prevalent among blacks in Harlem than among blacks in Africa.

One or more factors seem to be involved in the etiology of diverticulitis. The most widely held view is that a fiber-deficient diet is the principal cause of diverticulitis in the United States, northern Europe, and other highly developed countries with a long food pipeline from producer to consumer. This hypothesis is supported by the development of colonic diverticula in aging rats and rabbits fed diets unusually low in fiber.[4]

There is no clear-cut explanation for these findings but they were associated with the increased transit time and subsequent constipation observed with low-fiber diets.

Evidence that a low-fiber intake increases the incidence of colonic cancer is again mostly epidemiological and not as clear-cut as

Partial list of common drugs affecting vitamin levels in the elderly

Drug	Vitamin depleted	Comment
Mineral oil (found in many laxatives)	A,K,D	Chronic use results in these fat-soluble vitamins' elimination in feces.
Antibiotics	K	Some antibiotics destroy beneficial gut bacteria that produce K.
Isoniazid	B_6 (pyridoxine)	Long-term use of drug interferes with utilization of B_6.
Phenobarbital Phenytoin Primidone (Mysoline)	D	Especially for those on long-term anticonvulsant therapy.

that for diverticulitis.[4] Again multiple factors are probably involved in the etiology of cancer of the colon, but two dietary constituents are involved—low fiber and high fat.

At present, the most popular theory is that increased fat in feces is selective for a certain type of bacterium, providing a medium for the metabolic generation of low-grade carcinogens.[4] A diet low in fiber increases the time feces—and therefore low-grade carcinogens—remain in contact with the wall of the large bowel.

Fiber deficiency also leads to a reduced synthesis of bile salts so that their total concentration in bile is decreased. In addition, biliary concentrations of deoxycholic acid—a secondary bile acid formed in the intestinal tract by the action of bacteria on the primary bile acid, cholic acid—increases.

All of these processes are reversed by feeding bran, which removes the feedback inhibition of the primary bile acid chenodeoxycholic acid so that its concentration in bile rises. In turn, this rise stimulates the conversion of cholesterol to bile salts.[4] Thus, if bran is ingested in amounts no greater than those found in a natural diet, it will prevent or correct biliary lipid abnormalities believed to underlie the development of gallstones.

Diverticulitis, gallbladder disease, and cancer of the colon are costly in terms of mortality, morbidity, and health care. In 1967 the surgery alone to remove diseased gallbladders cost Americans about $500 million.[4] Added to this cost are financial losses due to time lost from work and premature death. At present, about $5 to $6 million is lost annually because of these diseases.

All of the evidence still isn't in on the relationship between nutrition and diverticulitis, gallbladder disease, and colonic cancer. However, the enormous cost in dollars and human suffering caused by these diseases demands immediate practical approaches to the problem, especially as the nutritional approach may have other benefits and no known contraindications, and may require only a minor change in life-style.

The kinds of changes I recommend are easy to incorporate in the cultural eating patterns of the elderly. They adhere to a somewhat unique eating pattern, according to recent studies, and their life-styles show a positive attitude toward health in general and toward food and eating. They're not faddists, but are willing to change at least some of their eating habits. They are not adverse to trying new foods, and they have good appetites. In fact, their eating habits and their selection of foods, including snacks, indicate that the elderly prefer foods with a high nutritional value. They dislike relatively few foods, and most eat three meals a day. Breakfast was the favorite meal for many.

As a population, therefore, the elderly are ideally suited to the kinds of nutritional changes I've recommended. Lean meat, fish, or poultry once daily, supplemented by skimmed milk and cheese, if they can tolerate them, will provide all of the protein and amino acids they require. Substituting margarine for butter, limiting the number of eggs eaten, and using low-saturated-fat products, reduces their intake of saturated fat. The fiber content of their diets can be increased by adding one or two tablespoons of bran to breakfast cereals—fortified cereals or other fortified products supply all the vitamin B_{12} and other vitamins needed. Red meats, liver, and certain fortified products provide needed iron. Calcium comes from milk and milk products, and any person who can't tolerate, drink, or eat them must take supplements.

These few simple dietary modifications will decrease some of the problems of your elderly patients, and, at the same time, delay diseases common to them.

References

1. Cristofalo VJ: A model system approach to the biology of aging. In *Nutrition and Aging* (Winick M, ed), ch 1. New York: Wiley, 1976
2. Masaro FJ: Physiologic changes with aging. In *Nutrition and Aging*, ch 4
3. Young VR, Perera WD, Winterer JC, et al: Protein and amino acid requirements of the elderly. In *Nutrition and Aging*, ch 5
4. Almay TP: The role of fiber in the diet. In *Nutrition and Aging*, ch 9

DATE DUE